Removable Denture Construction

Third edition

'Our objective should be the perpetual preservation of what remains rather than the meticulous restoration of what is missing'

M. M. De Van (1952) *J. Prosthetic Dentistry*, **2**, 210

Removable Denture Construction

Third edition

John F. Bates BDS, MSc, DDS, DrOdont
Emeritus Professor of Restorative Dentistry, Dental School, University of Wales College of Medicine, Heath, Cardiff, UK

Robin Huggett MSc, CGIA, FBIST
Special Lecturer and Chief Instructor, Dental School, University of Bristol, UK

G. D. Stafford TD, MSc, PhD, LDS, FDSRCS
Professor of Prosthetic Dentistry, Dental School, University of Wales College of Medicine, Heath, Cardiff, UK

WRIGHT
London Boston Singapore Sydney Toronto Wellington

Wright
An imprint of Butterworth–Heinemann Ltd
Westbury House, Bury Street, Guildford, Surrey GU2 5BH

 PART OF REED INTERNATIONAL P.L.C.

OXFORD   LONDON   GUILDFORD   BOSTON
MUNICH   NEW DELHI   SINGAPORE
SYDNEY   TOKYO   TORONTO   WELLINGTON

First published 1991

First published as *Removable Partial Denture Construction*
by John Wright and Sons, 1970
Second edition, 1978
Third edition published by Butterworth–Heinemann Ltd,
1991

British Library Cataloguing in Publication Data
Bates, John F. (John Frederick) 1924-
    Removable denture construction. — 3rd. ed.
    1. Man. Removable dentures. Design & construction
    I. Title.   II. Stafford, G. D. (George Derek)
    III. Huggett, R.
    617.692
    ISBN 0-7236-1667-1

Library of Congress Cataloging in Publication Data
Bates, John F.
    Removable denture construction/John F. Bates,
      Robin Huggett, G. D. Stafford. — 3rd ed.
        p.   cm.
    Rev. ed of: Removable partial denture construction.
      2nd ed. 1978.
    Includes bibliographical references and index.
    ISBN 0-7236-1667-1:
    1. Complete dentures — Laboratory manuals.
    2. Partial dentures — Laboratory manuals.
    3. Prosthodontics. I. Huggett, Robin.
    II. Stafford, G. D.   III. Bates, John F. Removable
      partial denture construction.   IV. Title.
    [DNLM: 1. Denture, Complete — laboratory
    manuals. 2. Denture, Partial — laboratory manuals.
      WU 25 M329p]
    RK656.B353   1991
    617.6'92 — dc20
    DNLM/DLD   90-13118
    for Library of Congress   CIP

Composition by Genesis Typesetting, Rochester, Kent
Printed in Great Britain at the University Press, Cambridge

Preface to the third edition

The dental student is usually introduced to clinical prosthetic dentistry by initially learning laboratory procedures associated with the production of various types of appliances. Without previous clinical experience, he/she finds it difficult to relate these procedures to the treatment of a patient. Most texts on clinical prosthetic dentistry do not have the laboratory procedure and clinical techniques in a logical order, and often appear unrelated so that the student of laboratory technology is easily confused.

Over the years the amount of time spent in teaching laboratory techniques has been reduced considerably and still constant pressure is brought to bear upon the dental teacher to reduce this time further. Every effort, therefore, must be made to ensure that the time available is used most efficiently.

The objective of this textbook is to provide the undergraduate and the student dental technician with enough clinical introductory material to explain the laboratory procedures and, at the same time, provide a logical sequence of steps in the construction of removable appliances. In the laboratory teaching of denture construction, complete denture procedures are easier to perform and less complex than partial denture procedures and are generally taught first. Thus, for this reason, we have presented laboratory complete denture construction prior to partial denture procedures. However, the first clinical case seen is usually partially dentate, so in presenting the clinical procedures we have presented the partial dentate stages first. This presentation format, which must involve some compromise, means that the complete denture clinical and laboratory stages run consecutively, but the clinical and laboratory partial denture stages are not consecutive.

Whilst the correct manipulation of the materials is specified, a discussion of dental materials has been left to the relevant applied dental materials textbook or to the references cited.

It is hoped, therefore, that this text will provide an introduction to laboratory and clinical practice during the first year of undergraduate teaching in the dental school. We also hope that it will be useful to dental technicians, dental hygienists and dental nurses who are interested in appreciating the problems of constructing appliances for patients.

Acknowledgements

We would like to thank our many colleagues who have helped with the preparation of this text by discussion, and suggestions of laboratory techniques. We thank the publishers Messrs Mosby for permission to utilize Figure 7.35 from Beresin and Schiesser's *The Neutral Zone in Complete Dentures,* and the Editor of the *Journal of Prosthetic Dentistry* for permission to publish Figure 7.33. To Professor Krol of the University of the Pacific, San Francisco we are indebted for Figure 8.10 and 10.8.

We must also acknowledge the invaluable help of our secretaries Mrs Glenys Williams, Mrs Zena Wright and Mrs Mary Hall for their patient work during the typing and correction of the manuscript, Mr Frank Hartles and his staff of the Visual Aids Department of the Dental School in Cardiff for the illustrations and Mr P. Sellen of Bristol Dental School.

Contents

1

Examination of the patient

Prosthetic treatment should be regarded as an approach to the solution of a patient's personal problem; and the first essential in solving the problem is to be in possession of all the facts. Success in prosthetic dentistry largely depends on the thoroughness of the preliminary examination, and treatment even of a simple kind should not be commenced before a thorough examination and diagnosis have been made.

Since patients are never exactly alike, it is necessary to find out by examination any individual peculiarities and difficulties, and only with this knowledge can subsequent procedures be adjusted to the optimum for the patient.

There are various ways of collecting the data; by visual examination, palpation or auscultation, tactile examination using probes, study casts, radiographs, by means of a history supplied by the patient, and from records of previous treatment.

The partially dentate patient

On the first visit it is essential to determine the patient's interest in dentistry and motivation towards retaining the teeth. This is not an easy assessment, since it does not relate to any factor which can be readily observed. For instance, it does not follow that for a person who is in the public eye and wishes to preserve teeth he is motivated to good oral hygiene. Research into the ability to educate adult patients in good oral hygiene habits has shown that it is extremely difficult to motivate patients into changing well established habits. Mature patients who have developed habits over many years find it difficult to change them. Occupation, marital status and social conditions are part of a patient's history and are important in assessing general behaviour.

The patient's complaint or reason for attending the dentist is also a useful indication of how dentistry is perceived and this, together with the patient's past dental experience, will be of assistance.

The method of taking a history and the examination of the patient is shown in Appendix I. In Appendix II the methods of assessing the periodontal condition and the amount of plaque on the teeth are described. The number of teeth missing and the number of restorations will also help to indicate how carefully the patient has looked after his teeth in the past.

The examination of the mouth also necessitates a scoring for tooth mobility. This is usually recorded on a scale from zero for no movement to three for movement greater than 2 mm in a horizontal direction together with axial movement. Scores of one and two are usually used for the amount of lateral movement in millimetres. The degree of attrition and the height of the teeth should be noted (Figure 1.1) and it is particularly important if crowns

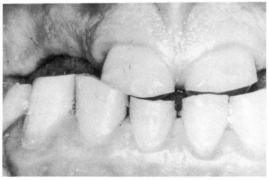

Figure 1.1 Attrition of the teeth

1

are to be made, since the retention is dependent on the length of the remaining preparation. Short crowns will give inadequate space if precision attachments are to be made and they will also provide poor guiding planes to help retention for a conventional denture. The length of the saddle area and the condition of the mucous membrane are important also, since, in a free-end saddle, the degree of movement will depend on the compressibility of the mucous membrane.

The occlusion should also be examined and an understanding of what is required to perfect the occlusion obtained. Study casts must be prepared and mounted on an articulator. This will assist in the process of any correction of the occlusion that might be necessary. This may be undertaken by grinding or use of onlays incorporated into the partial denture.

The occlusion

The examination should be performed in a systematic manner and the following mandibular reference points observed:

Retruded position (RP)

The retruded position of the mandible is the position of the mandible after maximal retrusion and can preferably be recorded when the first tooth contact occurs after a terminal hinge closure. This is generally referred to as the retruded contact

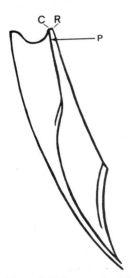

Figure 1.2 Movements of the mandible in the sagittal plane showing the retruded contact position (R) and the intercuspal position (C). The postural position is also shown (P)

position (RCP) which is synonymous with terms such as the ligamentous position or centric relation (Figure 1.2).

Muscular contact position (MCP)

The muscular contact position is the position when the occlusal surfaces have just reached contact after the mandible has closed with minimal muscle force and is synonymous with the terms centric occlusion and centric position.

Intercuspal position

Intercuspal position is the position of the mandible when the maximal occlusal contact occurs and is synonymous with habitual position or centric occlusion.

Postural position

The postural position (PP) is the position of the mandible when an individual is standing or sitting upright freely, is looking straight forward and when the masticatory muscles have minimal activity, and is synonymous with the term resting position.

During a functional examination of the occlusion it is important to observe the tooth contact in the retruded contact position and the intercuspal position and to note the gliding between these two positions.

Ideally, there should be even contact in the retruded contact position and the mandible should slide forward a distance not greater than 2 mm to the intercuspal position without lateral deviation.

If this does occur, then adjustment of the occlusion is essential and the treatment must be dependent upon examination of the study casts once they have been mounted.

In order to suppplement the knowledge of the periodontal condition and caries situation and to discover whether there are any pathological conditions which are not evident visually, it is essential to obtain radiographs. The ideal radiograph is an orthopantomogram (Figure 1.3) which demonstrates the whole of the dentition on the one film and does so with a minimum of radiation to the patient.

The edentulous patient

The examination of an edentulous patient must be carried out in a similar systematic manner and an 'aide memoire' in Appendix III sets out the approach to the patient and the areas to be examined. Initially, the same general information must be obtained as for a partially edentulous patient. The reasons for the patient needing the treatment and the past dental and past denture

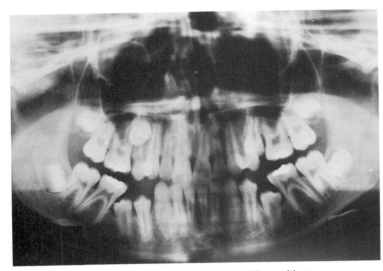

Figure 1.3 An orthopantomogram of the whole dentition and jaws

history are important in the complete denture wearer. Age is also important as the control of complete dentures requires considerable muscular coordination which is lost as one gets older. For those who have already worn dentures satisfactorily for some years this will not be a problem, but for the patient who is of an advanced age and been made edentulous recently, this may present considerable problems in learning to cooperate and to use the new appliance.

Patients with relevant medical problems and those on drug therapy will also have difficulties. Probably, the most important aspect in the examination is that of the details of the mouth, which is conducted with the objective of ascertaining the ability of the denture to resist displacement and obtain adequate support. Therefore, the size of the ridges and the depth of the sulcus (Figure 1.4), the thickness of the mucous membrane and the presence of sharp spicules of bone are of particular significance. A mucosa which is thin will not support the denture without pain and, likewise, an excessively thick flabby ridge (Figure 1.5) will allow the denture to move. Small or flat ridges (Figure 1.6) will not provide lateral stability and will thus allow the denture to move and become displaced.

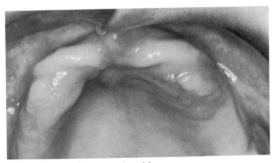

Figure 1.5 A flabby anterior ridge

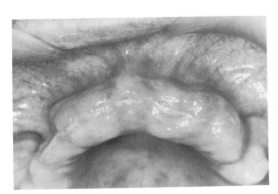

Figure 1.4 A patient with large ridges

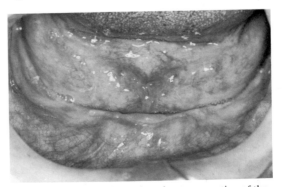

Figure 1.6 A very shallow sulcus due to resorption of the ridge which is now very reduced in size

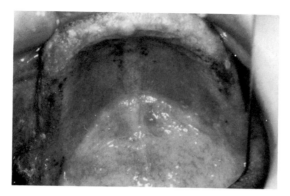

Figure 1.7 Candidiasis is probably the most common condition seen under complete upper dentures and covers part or whole of the denture-bearing area

For a denture to be retained in place, a fluid film is required between the mucosa and the denture and therefore the quantity and type of saliva is of importance, as is the mobility of the muscles. Some patients have very active musculature, whilst others have very little muscular movement during their speech and oral activity. Active movable tissues are more likely to displace dentures and will thus have considerable bearing on the ability of the patient to control the appliance.

Provided there is no pathology present in the mucous membranes, carrying out further investigations is not necessary, but if pathology is present, then this must be pursued by whatever method is most suitable (Figure 1.7).

The patient's personality and expectations are of considerable importance. Some patients are very

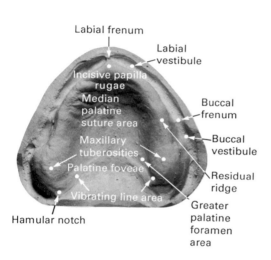

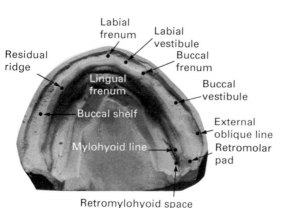

Figure 1.8 The anatomy of edentulous jaws

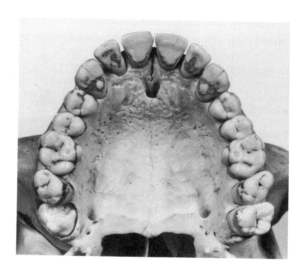

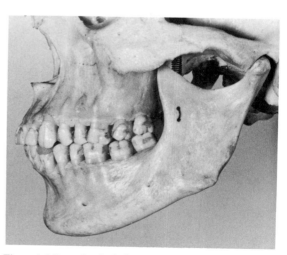

Figure 1.9 Dental articulation

exacting and demand perfection as they see it, whilst others are more placid and will collaborate easily to acquire competence with a satisfactory denture. It is important, therefore, to have a clear understanding of the patient's expectations of the denture and if very difficult patients have technically satisfactory dentures already, it may well be that they are impossible to satisfy. Remaking the dentures will only lead to further problems with the patient.

Careful assessment of the patient and the dentures will therefore guide the clinician to the appropriate treatment plan. This may involve modification of the existing dentures by, for example, relining or it may involve reconstructing the denture normally or using a modified technique such as duplication.

Figure 1.8 gives the anatomy of the jaws of an edentulous patient while Figure 1.9 indicates the dental articulation.

2

Preliminary impressions and occlusal records

Before the construction of any removable appliance can be undertaken it is essential to construct a cast of the patient's mouth in the laboratory.

The first procedure therefore is to take an impression of the patient's jaws using a material which will be fluid enough to flow into the small spaces and record the detail of the tissues but viscous enough to fill the tray and be capable of being conveyed into the patient's mouth. Once placed in the oral cavity the material must, by some means, be converted into either a rigid or elastic solid.

Table 2.1 lists the impression materials available together with some of their uses.

In order to convey the material into the mouth a tray is required. Trays are divided into two main groups, those which are mass produced to standard shapes by the commercial companies and those which are made individually for each patient – sometimes called custom-made or special trays.

The trays used will depend upon the clinical situation and will alter in shape depending on whether natural teeth are present or whether the patient is edentulous (Figure 2.1). Trays may be made from a number of different materials, such as stainless steel, aluminium or plastic and may be perforated to hold some elastic materials or be solid. The custom-made or special trays are always made from a plastic material which will be moulded to the shape of the cast of the patient's jaws. These latter custom-made or special trays are used for the final impressions for a patient.

The partially dentate patient

A manufactured dentate tray is used which should be modified by building up with impression compound in those places where the teeth have been

Table 2.1 Impression materials

Non-elastic	
Plaster of Paris	Seldom used as it fractures on removal from undercuts and casting is difficult.
Impression compound	Lower fusing used for preliminary complete denture impressions and in obtaining the periphery of impressions for complete dentures. Different colours indicate different melting points.
Zinc oxide–eugenol pastes	Two pastes when mixed give a smooth cream used for final complete denture impressions. Eugenol may be an irritant and has a short shelf-life.
Impression waxes	Mixtures of resins and waxes and gives a material which flows at mouth temperature, but must be cast immediately to prevent distortion and can easily be damaged.
Elastic	
(a) Hydrocolloids	
Reversible agar	Seldom used other than for crown and bridge restorations.
Irreversible alginates	The most common material for dentate and edentulous patients. Distorts easily and must be cast immediately due to water loss.
(b) Elastomers	
Polysulphides Silicones Polyethers	Widely used for partial denture impressions as storage is not a problem. Polyether and silicones are more difficult to bond to trays and perforated ones are essential. More expensive than alginates, but less likely to be distorted.

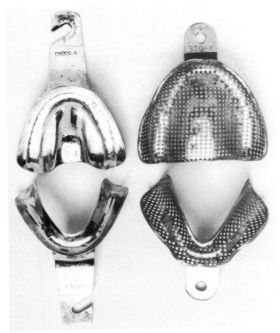

Figure 2.1 Perforated and non-perforated edentulous trays

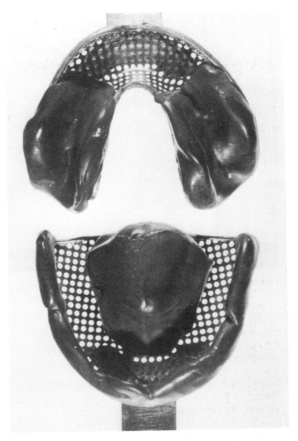

Figure 2.2 Perforated dentate trays modified with impression compound

extracted. This material is made in different colours depending on the softening point of the compound but for general purposes in this instance brown compound is used. This is heated to softening point in hot water until it can be kneaded with the fingers and placed in the tray. The tray is then inserted into the mouth after tempering and an impression is taken. On removal from the mouth, it may be necessary to trim off the excess material, cool the tray and then the compound will be coated with an adhesive material. The tray is then ready to take the definitive impression (Figure 2.2).

For preliminary impressions, the simplest and most commonly used material is an irreversible hydrocolloid. The material is mixed in accordance with the manufacturers' instructions, placed in the tray and inserted into the patient's mouth. In 3–4 minutes it will have set and be elastic and can be removed with a sharp snapping action. This is necessary due to the fact that rapid application of a force and release will cause less distortion in the impression material than a lower force applied for a long period. The tray and material is then washed and placed in a container which will prevent evaporation (100% relative humidity) (Figure 2.3). These materials lose water extremely rapidly and the impression must be taken into the laboratory and cast immediately.

Because of this problem, and where technicians are not always readily available, some practitioners use silicone materials. Softened modelling wax or a

soft wax may be moulded round the natural teeth and the tray is then loaded with a heavy-bodied (putty) material and an impression taken (Figure 2.4). A thinner mix of light-bodied material can then be coated on to the putty impression and when the wax is removed from the natural teeth this is again inserted into the patient's mouth and allowed to set. When withdrawn the more fluid light-bodied material will have recorded all the fine details of the oral tissues. When there are a number of natural teeth this technique is not very practical and it is preferable to mix the putty and coat it immediately with a light-bodied material and take a single impression (Figure 2.5). These impressions can be stored for some hours before casting but should preferably be cast the same day.

The facebow

The impressions which have been recorded will be poured to produce diagnostic casts and for partial

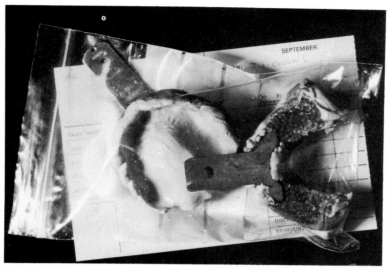

Figure 2.3 An impression in a container to keep it at 100% relative humidity

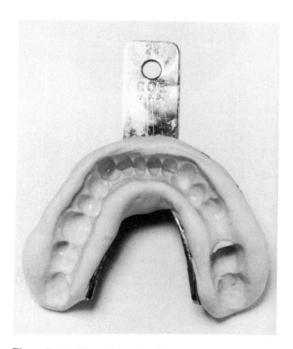

Figure 2.4 A silicone heavy-bodied impression

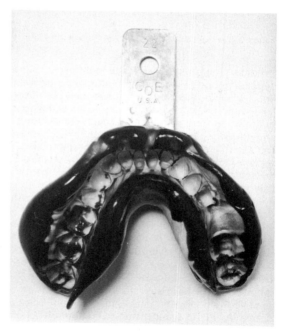

Figure 2.5 An impression corrected with light-bodied material

denture patients these need to be mounted onto an articulator for the occlusion to be studied. They must be positioned in the articulator the same distance from the joint mechanism as the natural teeth are from the condyle of the mandible and for this purpose a facebow is used (Figure 2.6). The facebow is taken together with an interocclusal record with the lower jaw in centric relation (Figure 2.7). The first stage of relating the facebow to the patient is to prepare, on the occlusal fork, a wax rim which can be softened and moulded to the upper teeth. This can then be lined with a zinc oxide paste

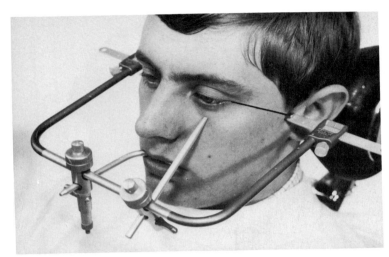

Figure 2.6 A facebow positioned on a patient

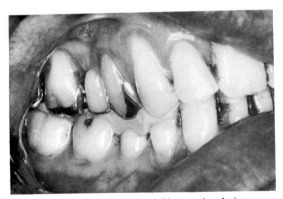

Figure 2.7 An interocclusal record in centric relation

to increase the accuracy if desired (Figure 2.8). It is also an advantage if the patient is asked to bite on the lower surface of the fork, thus maintaining the fork in a firm position in contact with the maxillary teeth. It must be emphasized that this is in no way a interocclusal jaw record.

A line is then drawn from the outer canthus of the eye to the superior edge of the tragus (Figure 2.9); 13 mm from the free edge of the tragus along this line a point is marked which, with the average patient, will be over the head of the condyle. For convenient application of the facebow it is best to pre-adjust the condylar rods symmetrically. Set one side to a fixed figure and leave the other side free. If the bow is then placed in position over the two marks representing the head of the condyle, the free end can be pushed in and the calibrated marking on its surface noted. The facebow is then removed and the two measurements on the rods are added

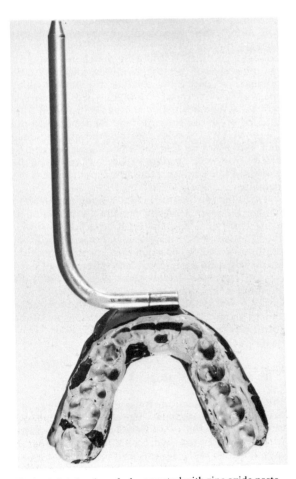

Figure 2.8 A facebow fork corrected with zinc oxide paste

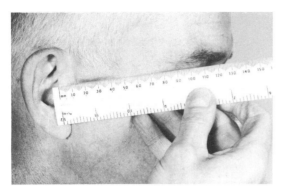

Figure 2.9 Marking the arbitrary position of the head of the condyle

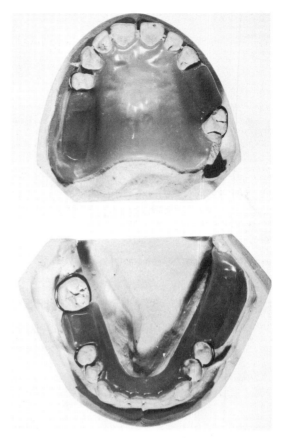

Figure 2.10 Occlusal rims for use in recording centric relation in dentate patients

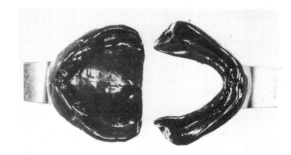

Figure 2.11 Compound impressions for an edentulous patient

together and divided by two. This will be the calibration marking to which each rod should be pre-set. For instance, if the fixed rod had a reading of 9 and on application to the face the other rod has a reading of 5.6, the total would be 14.6 and each rod should then be pre-set to 7.3. Re-apply the facebow placing it over the occlusal fork and it will be seen that the rods will lightly touch the two spots on either side of the face. With the rods over both points representing the condyle, the screw locking the bow to the occlusal fork is tightened. The orbital pointer is then positioned so that the tip is over the inferior border of the orbit and then locked to the facebow. The condylar rods can then be loosened and withdrawn so that the whole assembly can be lifted from the patient's face. Care must be exercised to ensure that the orbital pointer does not damage the patient's eye.

The mounting of study casts is often unnecessary if on examination of the patient the occlusion is satisfactory or if so many teeth have been lost that no occlusion posteriorly exists and only the anterior teeth are standing, or when one jaw is edentulous. In many cases, therefore, study casts do not need articulating. Also, if only some posterior teeth are present, it may not be possible to use an inter-occlusal record and occlusal rims will be required to obtain an accurate record of the relationship of the lower jaw to the maxilla (see Figure 2.10).

The edentulous patient

Preliminary impressions for complete dentures are taken either in compound, irreversible hydrocolloid or silicone. The latter is expensive and the majority of practitioners use hydrocolloid. If compound is used it can be replaced, renewed or added to until a satisfactory impression is recorded (Figure 2.11) which is an advantage in some cases. A wash impression inside the compound using a hydrocolloid or a light bodied silicone material is also often used particularly for difficult cases. A silicone putty impression with a light-bodied wash impression is also a common procedure.

Sterilization of impressions

Cross-infection between patient and technician can take place and ideally all impressions should be sterilized before being sent into the laboratory. In practice, this is a time-consuming procedure and for healthy patients not normally adhered to but with the spread of viral diseases such as hepatitis B and acquired immune deficiency disease (AIDS) it is becoming essential to sterilize all impressions for known carriers. Patients with undiagnosed viral diseases may still attend the practice and it is therefore an ideal procedure to sterilize all impressions. Appendix VII lists the precautions to be taken. Sterilization is obviously not an ideal treatment for hydrocolloid materials and it is for this reason that silicone impressions are now becoming widely used.

Communication with the laboratory

When the clinical procedures have been completed, it is essential that the wishes of the clinician are communicated to the technician. Clear written instructions or diagrams on work cards are mandatory and if there are difficult problems, discussion with the laboratory staff is always useful. If possible, the clinician should always draw the outline of trays on casts, but since few dental surgeons now have laboratories on the premises, this is not always a practical possibility and therefore, this places upon the technician a duty to understand the anatomy of the patient so that the trays will require little adjustment subsequently in the clinic.

Other factors which a clinician must decide and communicate to the laboratory staff are:

(1) The amount of spacing between the tray and the tissues required and the position of the stops to support the tray.
(2) Whether holes are required in the tray for retention.
(3) Position of the handle.
(4) The need for finger rests for the clinician to use when registering impressions.

Spacing is required when impression materials such as hydrocolloid are to be employed for the final impression since they tear easily and bulk must be provided around any natural teeth to prevent tearing as the impression is withdrawn. Usually a space is also provided over the edentulous areas.

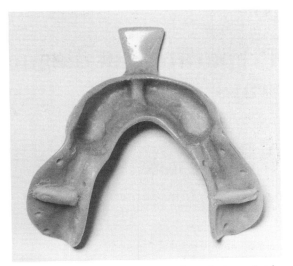

Figure 2.12 Stops in a special tray to keep the tray a fixed distance from the tissues

Spacing is always required around natural teeth for other materials also but since they are more tear resistant and provided they are elastic enough this spacing can be made smaller. For silicone and polysulphide materials relief over the edentulous areas can be very thin (0.5 mm) or may be omitted. Stops are provided to keep the tray in a stable position supported from the tissues whilst the impression material sets (Figure 2.12). The position of the stops will depend upon the position of the natural teeth.

Retention holes are generally only used for hydrocolloid materials although they can be helpful for silicone and polyether materials where the adhesives are not as reliable as with polysulphides.

The position of the handle will depend upon the individual tray. When natural anterior teeth are standing it can be parallel to the occlusal plane at the edge of the teeth, but in edentulous situations, it is better at right angles to the occlusal plane. It will then not interfere with lip movements whilst completing the final impression. When this information has been clearly transferred to the work card, the impression, facebow and records are sent to the laboratory.

3

Preparation of diagnostic casts and special trays

The casting of preliminary impressions represents the laboratory starting point in denture construction.

Diagnostic casts in complete denture construction

Diagnostic casts are also used for the construction of special trays and are poured in plaster of Paris which has adequate mechanical properties for this purpose. The upper and lower impressions are rinsed under cold running water and excess moisture is then removed by gently shaking or by gently blowing compressed air over the impression surface.

In a flexible mixing bowl 150 g of dental plaster per impression is mixed with cold tap water. The ratio will vary slightly with different batches of plaster. Approximately 40 ml water is required to 100 g plaster and so the water/powder ratio, will be approximately 1–2.5.

The plaster is gradually sifted into the water and mixed with a spatula ensuring as little air as possible is incorporated. Spatulation should continue until the mixture is of a smooth, creamy consistency. Care must be taken not to over-mix the material as this reduces the working and setting time.

Once mixed, the plaster can be gently vibrated into the impression. Avoid harsh or lengthy vibrations and handle the impression carefully. Place the impression on the mechanical vibrator and flow the plaster from one distal corner into the impression (Figure 3.1). Small increments of plaster are repeatedly placed in this region and allowed to flow over the impression surface. The impression is rotated whilst holding it against the vibrator moving the plaster slurry from place to place to ensure that no air is trapped. Gradually, more plaster is added

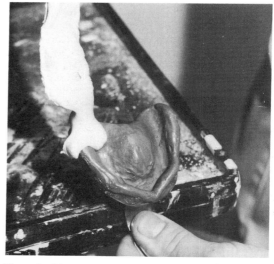

Figure 3.1 Plaster being poured into an edentulous impression whilst being vibrated to eliminate air entrapment

until the impression is completely filled. With compound impressions the remaining plaster in the bowl is placed on a tile or rubber mat and the impression inverted and gently seated on to it. The material is raked up the sides to form a base for the cast, being careful with the lower impression not to fill the space occupied by the tongue (Figure 3.2). When elastomers or hydrocolloid impressions are being poured it is preferable to allow the plaster in the impression to set before inverting it onto a mound of plaster to form the base.

As soon as the initial set has occurred in the plaster, the gross excess of material is trimmed away

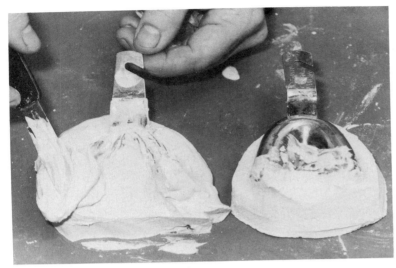

Figure 3.2 An impression based with plaster

from the sides and the cast made as neat as possible. When finally set (in approximately 30 minutes) the impression may be removed from the cast. Compound impressions are separated from the cast by placing the impression in hot water (60°C for approximately 6 minutes), when the compound will be thoroughly soft and can be carefully removed from the cast (Figure 3.3). Pieces of compound which adhere to the cast may be removed by pressing a piece of softened compound on to them – they will come away with it.

Alginate impressions should be removed from the cast within 1 hour as prolonged contact between the plaster and hydrocolloid results in a rough surface.

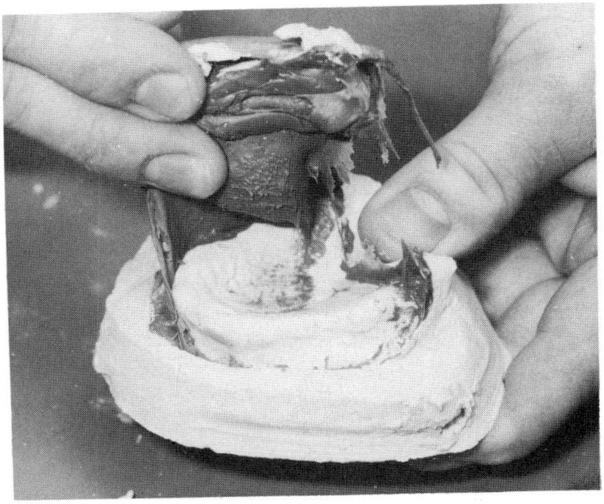

If adhesive materials have been used on the tray it will be necessary to remove the tray and impression in one piece and care must be exercised to ensure no damage is done to the cast. If a perforated tray has been used an adhesive is unnecessary and excess material from around the tray and the holes may be cut away and the tray separated from the impression material which can then be removed piecemeal.

Final trimming of the casts should be completed as soon as possible as any drying increases the hardness of the cast and makes trimming more difficult. Care must be exercised when trimming the side walls, as well as the base, to prevent damage to the anatomy of the cast especially in the tuberosity and retromolar pad areas.

The base of each cast is ground on the model trimmer (Figure 3.4) so that it is approximately parallel to the imagined plane of occlusion. The cast

Figure 3.3 Separation of the impression material from the cast

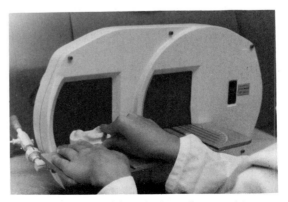

Figure 3.4 The base of the cast trimmed on a model trimmer to the finished state

should be approximately 1.5 cm thick at the thinnest point over the hard palate or tongue space. The sides of the cast are trimmed so that they are perpendicular to the base and to within 4 mm of the reflection of the sulcus tissues (Figure 3.4). This produces a land or art portion of the cast. The edges of the land area are bevelled downwards, using a sharp knife, to create a smooth border and, in the tongue area of the lower cast, the land area is also smoothed so that access to the lingual tissues can be obtained (Figure 3.5).

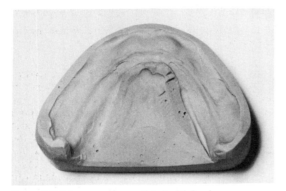

Figure 3.5 A lower cast completed with land area smoothed to give access to lingual borders

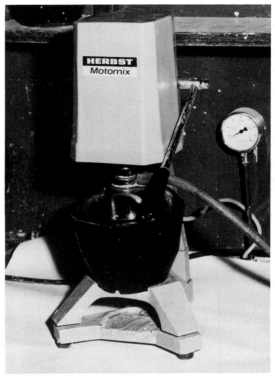

Figure 3.6 Vacuum mixing of stone for casts

Diagnostic casts in partial denture construction

The prime function of these casts in partial denture construction is to serve as a diagnostic aid and the construction is essentially the same as that described earlier. The impressions are generally taken in an irreversible hydrocolloid although silicone elastomers may be used. After the impressions have been removed from the mouth they should be rinsed with water and the excess moisture removed. Dental stone or die stone mixed with cold tap water in the water:powder ratio of approximately 1:3 is spatulated to produce a smooth mix. It has been shown that casts produced from mechanically spatulated stone are less porous than those produced by hand spatulation. The quality of the casts can be further improved by the removal of the trapped air using a vacuum at the time of mixing (Figure 3.6).

The stone slurry is poured slowly into the impression using vibration ensuring that no air is trapped into parts of the impression. Some support for the tray may be advisable to prevent the posterior borders of the impression from being distorted and on no account should the impression be inverted before the mix of stone has set as this

procedure may produce distortion of flexible impression material. The impression tray may be supported by the handle (Figure 3.7) to prevent the risk of distortion and the base is added later when the initial portion of the stone has set.

Once set, the impression should be removed from the cast. Care must be exercised as the teeth on the cast are easily broken and where possible the tray should be removed by freeing it from the impression material which can then be removed piecemeal. All positive surface nodules should be removed and the non-anatomical portion of the cast trimmed. Excess

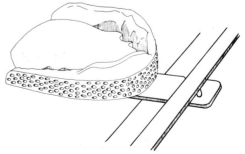

Figure 3.7 Tray supported prior to casting. The support is also used after the impression has been poured prior to basing

land on the cast can prevent them being correctly related to the centric occlusion record which will be discussed in Chapter 4.

The construction of special trays

A special or custom-made tray which is made specifically for an individual patient ensures that the impression material may be more accurately controlled by placing it and confining it to a specified area. Impression materials undergo a volume change during setting; the smaller the amount of material, therefore, the more accurate the impression. The special tray facilitates this and the impression is thus more accurate than the preliminary impression.

Special trays can be made from a variety of commercially available materials, including autopolymerizing acrylic resin, vacuum formed thermoplastic sheets of acrylic or polystyrene resin and shellac. It is important that the tray is rigid, uniform in thickness and that the method of construction is simple and economical. Only one method, that of constructing special trays from autopolymerizing acrylic resin, will be discussed in detail.

Complete dentures

The outline of the trays should be clearly drawn in pencil on to the diagnostic casts giving a clear pattern to follow, whilst fabricating and trimming the tray. When drawing the outline for the tray on the maxillary cast, particular attention should be given to the labial and buccal frenae. It is important that the outline of the tray is notched in these areas to avoid interference with fibrous or muscular insertions. Elsewhere, the outline should extend into the vestibule, staying approximately 2 mm above the tissue reflection, continue round the tuberosity region and proceed through the hamular notch and across the vibrating line area. The palatine foveae may or may not be visible on the casts. On the mandibular cast, the frenae should also be avoided. Elsewhere, the periphery should extend into the vestibule, on to the buccal shelves, across the retromolar pads and into the lingual sulcus of the mandibular arch, where it should be extended to the full depth of the sulcus (Figure 3.8).

Two kinds of special trays may be used in complete denture construction – close fitting or spaced.

Close fitting special trays

Those undercuts within the outlined area of the cast which would prevent the removal of the tray are blocked out with wax and the cast coated with a sodium alginate separating solution. The auto-

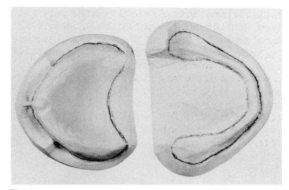

Figure 3.8 The outline of upper and lower special trays for complete dentures

polymerizing acrylic resin should be mixed according to the manufacturer's recommendations in conditions which will not endanger the health of the operator. The monomer should be measured into a porcelain or paper cup and the powder sifted into the liquid, spatulated and allowed to stand until the mass loses its sticky nature. Inhalation of monomer vapour can be dangerous and ideally mixing should be carried out in a cabinet with an extractor fan to the outside of the building or alternatively in a very well ventilated room. When the material has become a non-sticky dough and can be handled, it is either rolled or squeezed into a wafer of uniform thickness of approximately 3 mm. Monomer can penetrate the skin and create allergic responses or cause contact dermatitis and it is important for laboratory staff to protect the skin with a barrier cream or plastic gloves when handling the dough.

The acrylic resin wafer to be used for the upper cast is rounded and is shaped marginally larger than the upper cast (Figure 3.9). Wafers to be used for

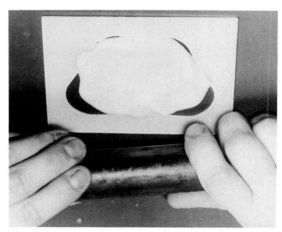

Figure 3.9 A wafer of autopolymerizing resin for tray construction

lower casts are prepared to a horse-shoe shape. The wafer is transferred to the cast and is pressed with light finger pressure to adapt it to the surface beyond the tray outline. The excess is trimmed away using a wax knife or scissors.

When hard, the rough tray can be removed from the cast and trimmed with stones and sandpaper until the periphery corresponds to the outline on the cast. Provided the material has been handled properly, the tray should need little smoothing (Figure 3.10) with burs and stones and is finally polished with pumice (see chapter 14 on polishing).

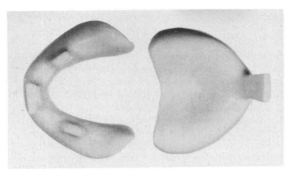

Figure 3.10 Completed trays in autopolymerizing resin prior to polishing

A small handle is placed vertically in the mid-line of the anterior region of both upper and lower trays. This configuration avoids interference with the lip. Two finger rests are placed in the second premolar region, on both sides of the lower tray. When the tray is used, these rests enable the operator to place the index fingers on the rests and position the tray without interfering in any way with the periphery of the impression (Figure 3.11). To add handles and finger rests, a small amount of acrylic resin is prepared to a dough consistency and moulded to the desired form. A monomer/polymer slurry is placed on the appropriate area of the tray and the undersurface of the handle or rest, and is then held *in situ* until polymerized.

Spaced trays

A spaced tray will be necessary where an elastic impression material is used to record substantial undercuts. The space allowed between tray and tissue should be sufficient and provide a uniform thickness of impression material for maximum accuracy and strength. The amount of thickness will vary depending upon the type of impression material used, as well as the amount of undercut present. To provide this space, modelling wax of the appropriate thickness is adapted to the area within the tray outline. A standard sheet of pink modelling wax is normally about 1.5 mm thick. Three small pieces are removed from the wax, one anteriorly in the midline and one each side of the molar regions (Figure 3.12). These small areas will appear in the tray as three raised areas or 'stops' which will then support the tray an even distance from the tissues.

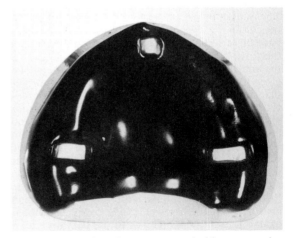

Figure 3.12 An edentulous cast covered with a wax spacing material. Parts of the wax have been removed to provide stops in the tray

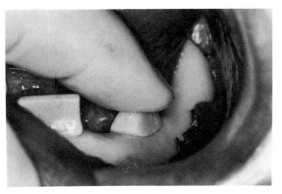

Figure 3.11 Finger rests preventing distortion of the periphery of the impression by the fingers

These locating stops will also impart stability to the seated tray and will lessen the risk of distortion in the impression due to movement of the tray during the setting of the material.

The autopolymerizing resin is mixed and the procedure for fabricating a spaced tray is the same as that described previously for close fitting trays.

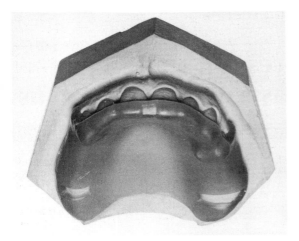

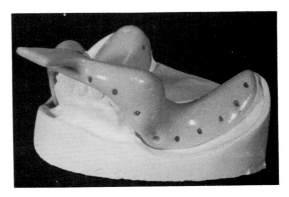

Figure 3.14 A tray, anteriorly showing the extension of the tray to only cover the incisal edges of the anterior teeth

Figure 3.13 A cast prepared for a spaced tray for a partial denture

Partial dentures

Spaced trays

For partial dentures the tray must be spaced round the teeth as the impression material must be free to disengage the undercuts associated with the teeth. The edentulous ridges may also be covered in 0.5 mm (casting) wax to create a small space under the tray. The amount of spacing is a personal decision of the clinician, which will depend on his decision as to the type of impression material used and the presence of undercuts. A similar procedure is adopted as for edentulous trays and the cast is covered in modelling wax (Figure 3.13) prior to the construction of the trays. The outline of the partial denture tray is modified to only include that area required for the construction of the appliance. For instance, there is no need for the sulcus depth to be recorded in those situations where the anterior teeth are standing (Figure 3.14). To do so would necessitate a greater force to displace the impression which may lead to inaccuracies. When the tray has been completed holes should now be drilled into the tray to act as retention for impression material.

4

Recording the final impression and preparation of master casts and occlusal rims

Recording the final impression

When the special trays are returned to the clinic/surgery it is necessary to ensure that they are cleaned to prevent cross-infection between laboratory staff and the patient. The simplest way of doing this is for the laboratory staff to place the trays in a sealed plastic bag containing a small amount of antiseptic solution such as glutaraldehyde (see Appendix VII). This will ensure that the plastic bag can be opened at the chairside in front of the patient. The tray can then be washed and is immediately ready for the operator to check in the patient's mouth that the extension of the tray is correct. It is becoming increasingly important that every effort must be made to ensure scrupulous cleanliness and that it is obvious to the patient that this is being done.

For partial dentures

Any adjustments to the tray are made to ensure that any over-extension which will prevent a correct final impression is removed and that any deficiency is corrected by the addition of compound or auto-polymerizing acrylic resin material to the tray. The periphery of the tray must be absolutely correct before proceeding to take the final impression. Once adjusted, the tray may be coated with an adhesive dependent upon the type of impression material being used (Figure 4.1). It is important that the adhesive be left for some time to dry as the success of an impression depends upon the rigidity of the tray and perfect adhesion between the material and the tray. If the impression can move on a semifluid adhesive the final impression will not be accurate. It is important that the tray only covers the area of the tissues required since extension of the

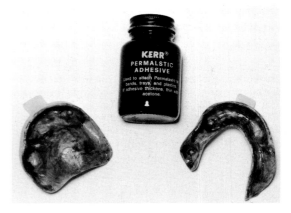

Figure 4.1 Adhesive applied to a tray for a partial denture and allowed to dry

tray to cover all the oral tissues will generate a suction effect when the tray is removed and thus a great deal more force will be required which will ultimately be applied at the material–tray interface and in some cases the adhesion will fail and an inaccurate impression will be produced. This will result in a metal partial denture which is inaccurate.

For complete dentures

Trays for the edentulous patient should be constructed with the periphery about 2 mm short of the actual reflection of the soft tissues. The clinician will then trace onto to the edge of the tray a softened material which will allow the patient to move his muscles and tissues and thus the tray will be peripherally moulded individually for each patient. The materials which can be used in this way are

Table 4.1 Materials used for the modification of the periphery of trays for complete denture impressions

Waxes	Korrecta wax	Four types of varying hardness. Care must be taken not to damage the wax when impressions are cast.
Compound	greensticks	Low melting point. Must be tempered correctly to obtain the best results.
Acrylic resins	butyl methacrylate-based materials	Long doughing and working times allow peripheral moulding before hardening.
Tissue conditioners	acrylic polymer, alcohol and plasticizer	Forms a gel which can be used for functional impressions over many hours.

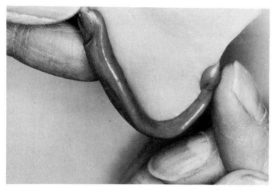

Figure 4.2 Greenstick tracing compound being applied to the periphery of a complete denture tray

listed in Table 4.1 but greenstick compound is a most satisfactory material (Figure 4.2). The whole of the periphery and the post-dam area of the tray is coated with the material, flamed with a torch and tempered in water at 55°C (Figure 4.3). The soft material can be adjusted in the mouth and moulded until the final impression will stay in place with a suction such as will occur with the final denture.

Once this has been achieved, the final impression material can be placed in the tray and a wash-like impression taken to achieve the recording of the fine detail. Since few edentulous impressions have undercut areas an elastic impression material is not essential and the most commonly employed material is a zinc oxide/eugenol impression paste. However, this is not a very clean material for handling in the

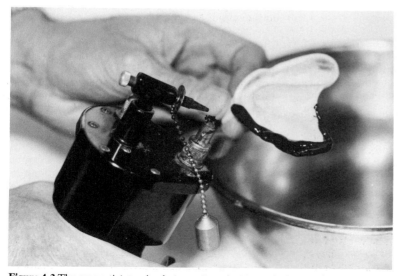

Figure 4.3 The greenstick tracing being softened with an alcohol torch

clinic or in the laboratory and many dentists now prefer to use silicone impression materials. The advantages of these, apart from the cleanliness, are that they can be easily sterilized in the same way as the preliminary impressions. Polysulphides are not as easy or clean to handle as silicones. Alginate materials are subject to absorption and dehydration in storage and sterilization is not easy.

Completion of design detail for the laboratory

Once the final impressions have been completed they are returned to the laboratory with the instructions on the work card for the subsequent laboratory procedures.

Metal partial dentures

It is important that the laboratory staff be given the design required by the clinician and therefore the work card should have a small printed section which includes a diagram of the teeth of upper and lower jaws upon which the design of the denture can be drawn. In addition, it is recommended that the design should be drawn on the study cast and if possible the use of different coloured pencils for the different parts of the denture should be used as this does help the laboratory staff to identify the design required. The type of alloy should also be specified and the amount of retention required on the various clasps and also whether autopolymerizing acrylic resin saddles are to be added to the framework prior to the denture being tried in the patient's mouth. The reason for this will become clear in Chapter 12.

Acrylic resin partial dentures

If an acrylic resin partial denture is to be constructed it will be essential, prior to the setting up of the teeth, that the relationship between the upper and lower jaws is recorded. It may well be that this may not be obvious from the natural teeth and therefore a temporary base with a wax occlusal rim will be required to record the relationship between the upper and lower jaws. In a similar manner to the metal partial denture the outline of the acrylic resin denture should be drawn on the work card and the laboratory staff will subsequently produce a base and occlusal rim to this shape.

Complete dentures

Since all the natural teeth have been removed the relationship between the upper and lower jaws is unknown. Before producing a denture it is necessary to ensure that this is known so that the two master casts can be transferred onto an articulator in the laboratory reproducing the correct relationship of the jaws.

In the adult person with natural teeth a small space exists between the the teeth when at rest. The height of the face in this position is called the resting face height and when the jaw is closed and the teeth come into contact the face height is called the occlusal face height. The difference between these two measurements is 2 to 3 mm and is called the freeway space. When the natural teeth are extracted, there is little change in the resting face height and this therefore acts as a base line from which the height of the artificial teeth can be assessed. When the dentures are inserted there should therefore be a 2–3 mm space between them when the patient is relaxed.

Likewise, when the natural teeth are together the horizontal relationship between the maxilla and the mandible is one where the temporomandibular joint is in its most retruded unstrained position and this is often referred to by a number of different terms, i.e. centric relation, muscular contact position and should be coincident with the centric occlusion of the natural or artificial teeth. The objective of the next stage of treatment, therefore, is to produce a base exactly like the denture base upon which wax rims are placed to represent the artificial teeth. These rims can then be adjusted and the correct jaw position recorded.

When the final impressions are transferred to the laboratory, instructions must therefore be given regarding the design of the bases and the rims to be used at the next clinical stage. For the majority of cases, the bases are temporary and constructed in wax, shellac or autopolymerizing acrylic resin. Wax rims are then added to these but in some instances a final denture base in heat cured acrylic resin is made on the master cast to which the wax rims are added. The master cast is thus destroyed in this process as it will not be needed again and the artificial teeth are either heat polymerized or autopolymerized on to this master base. This has some advantages in ensuring a well fitting retentive denture base which aids in the recording of accurate jaw relationships. *Also rigid + stable at mouth to.*

Reference to the notes on retention in the appendix will make it clear that to prevent the flow of saliva under the denture a seal is required at the posterior border of the upper denture. This can be achieved by pressing the tissues whilst the impression is recorded but it is more common to scrape a trough on the cast (Figure 4.4). This post-dam is best carried out by the dental surgeon but in many instances, it will have to be produced in the laboratory. It must be emphasized that to achieve the optimum retention of the bases it must be produced before constructing the base for the occlusal rims.

Reason for acrylic base

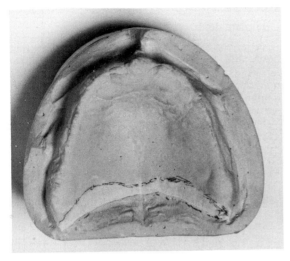

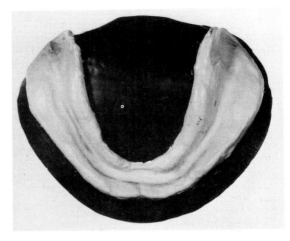

Figure 4.5 A lower cast beaded prior to casting

Figure 4.4 A cast in which the post-dam has been prepared

Laboratory stages

Preparation of master casts

The final impressions are probably the most important recordings sent to the laboratory. The master cast is a detailed reproduction of the patient's teeth and tissues. This cast is of paramount importance, its accuracy will determine the stability and the retentiveness of the denture and is essential to patient comfort and satisfaction.

In complete denture construction

Final impressions are beaded and sometimes boxed with wax. This helps to obtain and preserve a reproduction of the border of the impression. Soft beading wax, approximately 5 mm wide, is attached around the periphery of the impression 3 mm below and parallel to the border. In lower impressions the lingual area is filled with conventional modelling wax (Figure 4.5). This beading of the impression ensures the important sulcus area is reproduced to the full extent of the reflection and is protected by an adequate width of stone. In addition, boxing or modelling wax may then be attached to the beading to build side walls against the beading to provide a base into which the stone can be vibrated (Figure 4.6), although this later stage is not always considered necessary.

The final impressions are poured in stone following the same procedure as that used for preliminary impressions described in detail earlier.

The stone is mixed (ratio 1:3) and vibrated slowly into the anatomical part of the impression and onto the wax beading until the impression is full (Figure

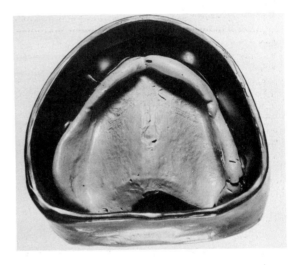

Figure 4.6 Boxing in an upper impression

4.7). When non-elastic type impression materials have been used, the poured impression may be inverted onto a mound of the stone mix. With elastic type impression materials the two-stage procedure described earlier is used. When the initial set of the stone takes place excess material may be removed.

Approximately 1 hour is allowed for the stone to set before removing the impression material. The beading/boxing wax is peeled away first. After the wax has been removed, the stone master casts and impression are placed in a bowl of hot water (60°C) for 4 minutes. The compound border moulding will soften and the tray may be released from the cast. A

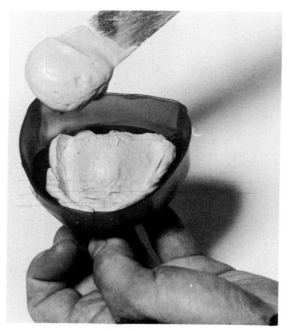

Figure 4.7 Casting the final impression

knife is used to gently pry the impression tray off of the master cast being careful that no damage takes place.

The bases of the casts are trimmed so that they are parallel to the imagined plane of occlusion and 1.5 cm thick at their thinnest point. The sides of the cast should be trimmed at right angles to the base leaving a border of about 5 mm to protect the margins formed by the impression.

In partial denture construction

The preparation of these casts is a variation of the procedures already described but some laboratories prefer to use die stones rather than ordinary dental stone to ensure that the casts have maximum hardness and abrasion resistance. However, in beading the elastomer type of materials, it is often found that the beading wax will not readily adhere to the impression material and sticky wax must first be applied to the impression to provide an interface for the beading wax. With some silicone materials, where even sticky wax will not adhere, then the first stage of preparing the cast, the pouring of the anatomical portion, must be built up carefully to ensure that the peripheral borders are well covered with an adequate thickness of stone. When this first part has set and the base is added, it is important to ensure that there is adequate support for the vital sulcus areas.

Occlusal rim construction

Complete dentures

A variety of materials may be used for constructing bases and rims. The most common material is modelling wax for both base and rim. Other materials used are shellac, often reinforced with aluminium powder, vacuum formed polystyrene sheet or autopolymerizing acrylic resin.

The most commonly used combination of materials is the use of a wax base and rim. Its advantage over other combinations is its ease and speed of construction, together with lower material costs. The main disadvantage of the all-wax assembly is that the base may soften at mouth temperature, which could lead to distortion, thus making recording difficult and possibly causing an error in the record. A good quality toughened wax reduces the possibility of this error.

The construction of the base

Before constructing the base a post-dam should be cut in the upper cast. Some clinicians, when taking the impressions, achieve this by exerting pressure on the impression as it sets. In the majority of cases, however, modification of the cast is essential and this is shown in Figure 4.4. The cast is scraped with a wax knife to give the required shape and depth.

Construction procedure

Wax base A separator such as french chalk or microfilm is applied to the cast and sufficient modelling wax to cover the cast is softened over a bunsen burner or in hot water and adapted to the cast. The palate or lingual aspect is adapted first, and this is held firmly in place whilst the wax is closely adapted to the buccal and labial aspects. The wax is trimmed to the peripheral edge of the sulcus and to the palatal finishing line by use of a warm wax knife.

A wire strengthener, (e.g. 1.0 mm dia. soft nickel silver) is bent to approximate the lingual or palatal contour of the alveolar ridge. Its length is trimmed to end at the medial edges of the retromolar pads or tuberosities. The wire strengthener is warmed and placed in position in the wax base so that its top edge is about 2 mm below the crest of the ridge. It is sealed in position with molten modelling wax. A prepared wax base is shown in Figure 4.8.

Softened wax is added to the concavity of the sulcus area and light finger pressure applied to minimize distortion. The base is removed from the cast, its fitting surface checked for accuracy of detail and sharp edges removed before returning the wax base to the cast.

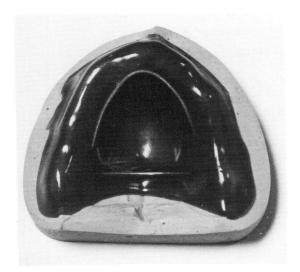

Figure 4.8 Wire strengtheners in a wax base prior to the construction of the occlusal rim.

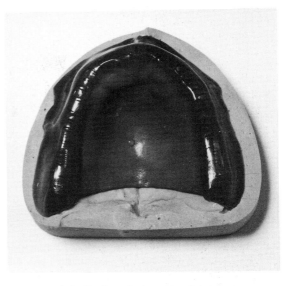

Figure 4.9 A shellac base for an occlusal rim

Shellac base Shellac is more difficult to manipulate than wax and must be quickly moulded as it hardens rapidly. When hard, it is extremely brittle but provides a rigid base that is more stable than wax at mouth temperature.

Any undercut areas that might cause the rigid shellac base plate to lock onto the master cast are blocked out with wax. (If undercut areas are very extensive and severe it might be advisable, after 'blocking out' to duplicate the cast and construct the shellac base on the duplicate.)

The cast is soaked in water to prevent sticking of the base plate. The shellac base plate is softened over a bunsen flame or is placed upon the cast and the flame brushed across the surface. When soft the shellac is adapted to fit the cast, care being taken to avoid thinning or overheating the base plate. The excess base plate material that extends over the land of the master cast can be cut away with scissors while the material is soft. After gross trimming, the base plate must be closely trimmed to fit the master cast. This final shaping and trimming may be accomplished by using a rotary cutter or by the use of a file. The base plate may need further heating and adaption before the edges are finally smoothed with sandpaper (Figure 4.9).

An autopolymerizing acrylic resin base Undercut areas on the cast must be blocked out with wax and the cast coated with an alginate separating solution. The base made be moulded by adapting the autopolymerizing acrylic resin, at the dough stage to the cast in the same way as that described in the previous chapter for special tray construction.

Alternativly this can be built up on the cast by applying liquid monomer to the cast and sprinkling polymer powder into the liquid. Repeated application of monomer and polymer onto the cast will gradually build up the base to the required thickness. It is essential that this technique is carried out in a special ventilation cabinet to prevent inhalation of monomer vapour.

Polymerization of the autopolymerizing base plate will take approximately 20 minutes. This stage may be quickened and the properties of the material enhanced by placing the cast and base into a pressure curing pot (Figure 4.10) in warm water for approximately 30 minutes at 35°C and pressure of 2.2 bar. The baseplate is smoothed and finished as

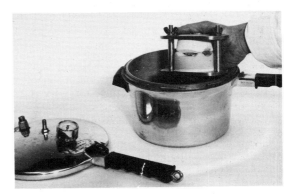

Figure 4.10 A pressure pot/Polyclav/Hydroflask for curing autopolymerizing resin

previously described for finishing special trays and the base can then be fitted to the master cast prior to the construction of the occlusal rim.

Permanent acrylic resin base (heat cured) Heat-cured acrylic permanent bases are sometimes used with occlusal rims. After the occlusal recordings have been taken, the bases are used for the try-in stage and the teeth are finally processed to these bases to form the completed dentures. Heat-cured bases as well as being rigid and stable at mouth temperature, also enable a check on the accuracy of the final impressions to be made, and provide retention and stability that should be equal to that of the finished denture.

A wax base to the required thickness is prepared on the master cast and sealed down around the edges ensuring that the full depth and width of the sulci of the cast are filled. The flasking procedure follows that recommended for complete dentures (Chapter 14). The baseplate may be constructed in either clear or coloured acrylic resin. The clear acrylic resin is often preferred as it may permit any discrepancies of pressure on the mucosa to be visible. When deflasked the peripheries and non-fitting surfaces are smoothed and polished. The procedure is the same as that described for complete dentures (Chapter 15).

The master cast is usually destroyed when the acrylic base is deflasked after processing. As a cast is required for the subsequent rim construction and try-in stages it is necessary, using plaster of Paris, to pour a keeper or working cast into the acrylic base after blocking out any undercuts with modelling wax.

The construction of occlusal rims

The rims are made of wax. The wax rims can either be fashioned from sheet wax or preformed rims may be used. There is no doubt that the preformed rims save considerable time and are more homogeneous.

The occlusal rims should be fixed firmly to their bases. The lower rim should lie directly over the crest of the residual ridge and extend to the area of the first molar on each side.

The upper rim should be positioned over the crest of the residual ridge posteriorly, stopping short of the tuberosities. In the anterior region, it should be positioned so that its labial surface reproduces the original contour of the labial surfaces of the natural anterior teeth, which is approximately 8–10 mm forward of the incisive papilla.

The height of the upper rim is shown in Figure 4.11. The upper rim height measurement from the mucolabial fold adjacent to the frenum to the occlusal plane level should be 22 mm and the lower rim 16 mm; the average overall height of both rims totalling 38 mm. The upper rim should decrease in

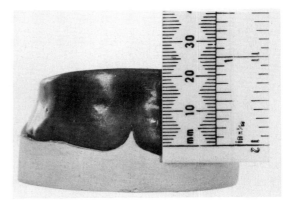

Figure 4.11 Occlusal rims for an edentulous patient

height from the anterior region until the area of the last molar is 7–8 mm above the centre of the alveolar ridge. The lower rim should be gradually reduced to the level of the retromolar pads.

When the wax rims have been trimmed to conform to the required measurement, the sides are trimmed (or built up) and smoothed to produce a contour that flows to the sulci or palate. Distal to the first molar region, the upper rim should slope at approximately 45° to the end of the tuberosities.

Whilst the sizes of the rims stated are average ones the technician must observe the anatomical points which are evident on the cast and construct the rims accordingly. For instance the retromolar pad lies, as its name implies, behind the third molar tooth in the natural dentition and the height of the occlusal rim should therefore be no higher than the mid point of this pad (Figure 4.12). Generally there is also a line of soft tissue remaining after the extraction of the upper teeth which is the remainder of the palatal gingivae and this can be seen on most

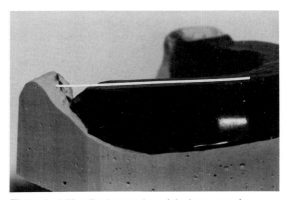

Figure 4.12 The distal extension of the base onto the anterior half of the retromolar pad

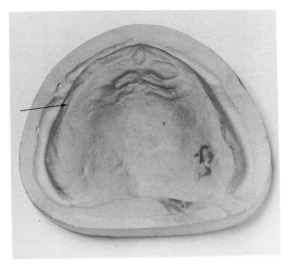

Figure 4.13 Remnants of the palatal gingivae in the maxilla

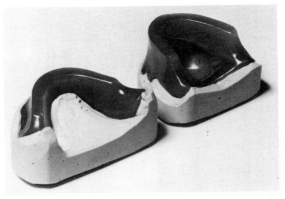

Figure 4.14 The rim as it passes from the occlusal surface to the sulcus is concave in shape

casts (Figure 4.13) and the rims should be set buccally to this line.

The occlusal rims should not be bulky and should be reduced as much as possible to avoid constricting the tongue. A concave curved shape from the occlusal surface to the sulcus will harmonize with the oral musculature and aid retention (Figure 4.14).

The rim and base assembly are removed from the cast and the outer edge of the periphery of the base smoothed without damaging its contour. The assembly is returned to the cast.

Finally, the occlusal rims are given a gloss by flaming, followed by rubbing with cotton wool, whilst held under cold running water. A small amount of soap on the cotton wool enhances the finished appearance and is an aid to cleanliness.

Partial dentures

Base construction and occlusal rims for partial dentures

In partial denture construction, if insufficient teeth are present it may be necessary to construct occlusal rims. Occlusal rims used to obtain a record of centric occlusion are shown in Figure 2.10.

Essentially, the techniques of construction of partial occlusal rims are the same as are used in complete denture construction. The bases of the occlusal rims are usually constructed from either wax or shellac and they are made to finish above the survey line of standing teeth in the posterior region and to rest on the cingulum of the anterior teeth. The wax rims should be placed in the edentulous saddle areas contacting the abutment teeth. The standing teeth are used as a guide for the rim's dimensions. The rim should not protrude above the occlusal surface of standing teeth, or be wider than them. They should be trimmed and positioned to fill the space of the teeth they are replacing. Finishing of the rims follows the method previously described.

5

The recording of jaw relationships in edentulous patients

In the previous chapter an explanation of the need for trial bases and occlusal rims was given. This chapter provides a brief description of the clinical procedures which are necessary for the next stage of complete denture construction. This procedure involves registering the relationship of the lower jaw to the upper in both vertical and horizontal directions.

The rest position

Before the clinical procedures can be understood it is essential to appreciate the anatomical and physiological factors affecting the positions of the jaws. When the natural teeth are present, the muscles normally have an essential activity which controls their length and when the natural teeth are extracted the length of the muscles remains much the same although they will be affected since the weight of the lower jaw will have been reduced which will cause some gravitational change. However, for practical purposes we can assume they remain the same length and as a guide to obtaining the occlusal vertical dimension it is presumed that no change takes place when the natural teeth are removed.

It is of the utmost importance in denture construction that the height of the artificial dentures does not interfere with muscle activity, and that mastication, swallowing and speech are not impeded. The selection of a suitable height for the dentures depends on the assumption that when the patient is relaxed and the lower jaw at rest the muscle length remains constant. In this position, called the rest position, the natural teeth will have a slight space (the freeway space or interocclusal space) between them. As the elevator muscles contract and the depressor muscles relax, the mandible will be raised and the teeth will be brought into occlusion. This cannot be maintained for long periods and eventually the muscles will relax and the jaw return to the resting position when all the muscles attached to the mandible will remain in equilibrium. Gravity and body position will, however, affect this as does individual jaw relationships. Therefore, when no teeth are present if the resting position can be established the occlusal height of the denture can be attained by reducing the height by 2–4 mm.

Since it is impracticable to measure inside the mouth, these measurements are established on the outer part of the face (Figure 5.1).

Resting face height − (2–4) mm = occlusal face height

The retruded jaw position

Having obtained a means of establishing the vertical dimension of the dentures it is now also important to consider the horizontal relationships. The jaw position is controlled to a very fine degree by proprioceptors in the temporomandibular joint muscles, the periodontal ligaments of the teeth and also the soft tissues of the oral cavity. This enables the patient to close successfully in the same position where all the teeth will intercuspate (centric occlusion). When the teeth are lost a considerable amount of proprioceptive feedback is also lost and it is therefore important to obtain a jaw recording so that the patient can repeat the same procedure with the artificial dentition and close dentures together into centric occlusion. Failure to do so will lead to the dentures moving on the soft tissues under the denture and cause soreness.

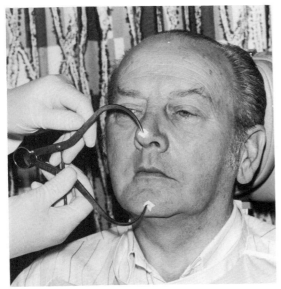

Figure 5.1 Measuring facial dimensions

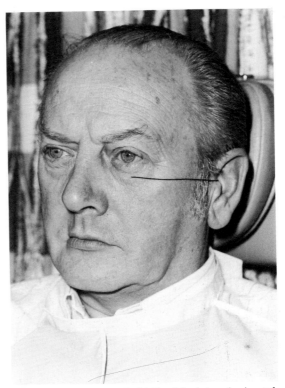

Figure 5.2 Patient seated with Frankfurt plane horizontal

When the natural teeth are in centric occlusion, both the temporomandibular joints will be in their most retruded, unstrained position and the mandible is said to be in centric jaw relationship. It is essential to record this position with the occlusal rims at the agreed vertical dimension. More retruded positions of the temporomandibular joint can be obtained provided force is applied to the mandible and the lateral ligaments of the joints strained but this is not a natural position for the jaw and it is not a desirable position to record. Provided the temporomandibular joints are in their most retruded position the mandible cannot deviate laterally, thus it will be possible to record with the occlusal rims and bases a three-dimensional relationship of the mandible to the maxilla which will then be transferred to the articulator in the laboratory.

Clinical procedure

Like the special trays, the trial bases and occlusal rims should be returned to the clinic in a plastic bag containing disinfectant. Alternatively, they should be soaked prior to use and placed in a prominent position on the bracket table. The patient will be seated in an upright position such that the Frankfurt plane is horizontal (Figure 5.2).

Stage I

The bases are placed in the patient's mouth and checked for retention and stability. If permanent bases are used the retention and stability should be

as good as can be obtained from a complete denture but where trial bases are used these are seldom as retentive, but they should be adequate and ensure satisfactory retention and stability when the denture is completed. If retention is not satisfactory at this stage this must be corrected once the fault has been determined and it may necessitate taking new impressions if the casts are inadequate.

Stage II

Lip support The patient is observed in profile in order to assess the amount of lip support which will be necessary from the denture. The lips should show a reasonable amount of vermilion border when the upper rim is in place. This however will depend to a large extent on the patient's age and previous denture experience and may also depend on the patient's wishes with regard to aesthetics. Many dentures are made with inadequate lip support and with time the lip contracts and it may therefore not be possible to support the lip in exactly the same way that it was supported with the natural teeth although this would be the ideal. The support of the lip depends on the labial surfaces of the artificial teeth and in a normal jaw relationship the labial surfaces are at an angle of 108° to the Frankfurt plane and thus the labial face of the occlusal rim should be trimmed accordingly.

The occlusal rims are the 'prescription' to the technician for setting up the teeth and great care should be taken to ensure that the contours of the occlusal rims are correct as eventually the position of the teeth will affect speech.

Neutral zone The stability of the denture will also depend on the position of the artificial teeth in relation to the muscles of the lips and cheeks on one side and the tongue on the other. The neutral zone is a concept which relates to the natural dentition and is the area in which the natural teeth lie between the muscles and soft tissue on each side of them.

Both these muscle masses during activity cause pressure to be applied to the teeth and their eventual position occurs because the forces cause equal effects and the teeth become stabilized in that area. Whilst the artificial denture can not be related to the neutral zone the concept is useful and the artificial teeth should lie in an area of minimal muscle activity.

This will be checked more carefully at the trial stage.

Stage III

The height of the occlusal plane The upper rim is adjusted so that the lower border of the rim represents the tips of the incisor teeth which will vary with individual lip length but in 'normal' circumstances and in young people 1 mm is an average amount of tooth showing below the the lip at rest.

The rim is then made parallel to Camper's plane which is a plane formed by joining the naso-labial-tragus lines on each side of the face (Figure 5.3).

Stage IV

Assessing the resting vertical dimension The upper base and the occlusal rim are placed in the patient's mouth and the patient is asked to relax and sit as quietly as possible. Considerable variation exists due to patient nervousness at the feeling of a strange object in his/her mouth. A number of methods may be used to help the patient, such as swallowing and relaxing, saying the letter M and also licking his lips.

It is not possible to measure intra-orally and therefore the measurements are made on the patient's face and two methods are commonly employed. One is to use a measuring gauge such as the Willis gauge (Figure 5.4) or, alternatively the use of marks on the patient's face and calipers (Figure 5.1). When it is felt that the mandible is in the rest position and it is possible to reproduce the

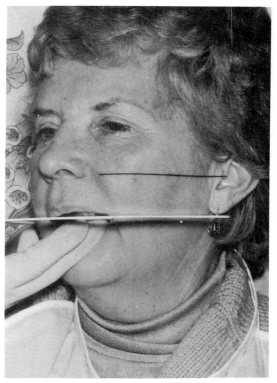

Figure 5.3 A Fox guide plane to ensure that the occlusal rim is parallel to Camper's plane

position on a number of occasions, the measurement obtained by the calipers or the Willis gauge is the resting vertical dimension.

Stage V

The establishment of the occlusal vertical dimension The upper and lower bases and rims are inserted in the mouth and the jaws closed. It will be seen by how much the lower rim must be adjusted to allow the two rims to close together in even contact. The lower rim is then softened and trimmed until even contact is achieved and the facial measurements are then retaken. This is repeated with further adjustments in the height of the lower rim until the occlusal vertical dimension is 2–4 mm less than the resting dimension. When this stage is reached, the patient should be able to relax and can tell that a small space exists between the rims or by parting the lips carefully, the operator can also observe that the rims are not in contact.

Errors arise if the rims contact prematurely at the posterior area of the jaw as the anterior part of the rim will then be lifted up and the rim will appear to be in even contact. Even if the base is not displaced

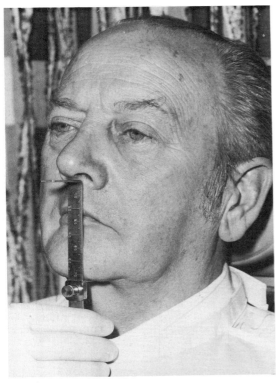

Figure 5.4 Willis gauge to assess facial dimensions

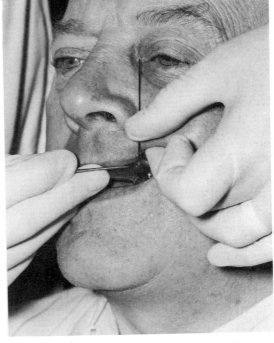

Figure 5.5 Marking the canine lines on the occlusal rim

uneven compression of the soft tissue will lead to inaccuracies in the recording. It is wise therefore to ensure that the bases are not in contact and that this can be checked by passing a blunt probe between the rear parts of the bases.

The technician setting the artificial teeth will need to know the centre of the patient's face and thus a centre line must be recorded on the wax rims. The best guide to this is the labial frenum, but because few patients' faces are symmetrical, this must be decided on the aesthetics required.

The length of the upper lip varies greatly in patients and the height to which it will rise when smiling varies and to help with the setting of the teeth this must also be marked on the wax rim.

Two canine lines should also be marked. These are vertical lines which pass from the tip of the canine to the alar of the nose and the inner canthus of the eye (Figure 5.5).

Stage VI

Recording centric jaw relationship The patient should now be able to open and close the jaws in comfort and the next stage is the recording of the position of the lower jaw in its most retruded

position. Only the most retruded position is reproducible and thus the jaw relationship is practised until reproducibility is obtained. Two lines may be scored in the premolar area through the upper and lower rims when the position is established. The scored lines in the mid line and in the lateral regions can be useful since repeated attempts to obtain the retruded position will show that the lines always coincide.

A number of techniques are used to obtain the most retruded position. They are as follows:

(1) Curling the tongue back to touch the posterior part of the upper plate.
(2) Asking the patient to swallow.
(3) Clenching the rims together and ensuring that the anterior temporalis muscles are contracted.
(4) Ensuring that the jaw is relaxed and guiding it with the fingers along a rotational movement until contact is achieved. If the patient attempts to push the lower jaw forward the operator will be able to feel this and with further practice the sensation of rotation of the jaw can be felt (Figure 5.6).

Once this position has been noted and the lines coincide the upper rim is notched and the lower

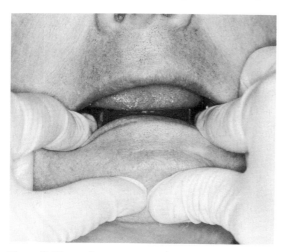

Figure 5.6 Recording centric jaw relation

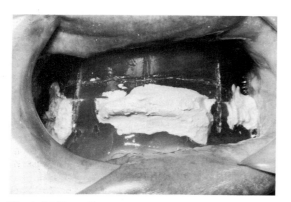

Figure 5.7 Recording centric jaw relation

reduced leaving two pillars in the premolar regions where the score marks have been made (Figure 5.7). Quick setting impression plaster, silicone or zinc oxide paste can then be coated on to the lower rim which is then inserted and the retruded position established again. The patient is then allowed to sit in this position until the material has set and the lower jaw should be supported by the operator.

The advantage of using a soft material to record the position ensures that there is no displacement of the bases or undue compression of the underlying soft tissue. With these fluid materials it may be difficult to ensure that the patient remains in a static position for long enough for the material to set. If this does occur then softened wax can be used instead and on closure cold water can be sprayed on to the wax to cause it to harden. Waxes tend to soften in the laboratory and care must be taken to prevent inaccuracies by mounting the cast as soon as possible.

The gothic arch tracing

The simple hinge opening and closing of the jaw when the condyles are in the most retruded position with the jaw muscles relaxed, is the technique generally employed for recording centric jaw relationship. However, in some cases patients find it almost impossible to undertake this relaxed movement and a gothic arch tracing device is a technique which assists in overcoming this. It is, however, time consuming and it is only employed in difficult cases. Gothic arch tracing devices are intra-oral or extra-oral (Figure 5.8) but both require a centre bearing point fitted into the bases at the correct occlusal vertical dimension (Figure 5.9). In intra-oral devices this centre bearing point is a pointed screw for carrying out the actual recording. The principle of these devices is that when the jaw moves from side to side the condyles rotate alternately and the jaw thus swings around one condyle. The marking device thus records this movement and travels on an arc, the centre of which is the condyle. The arcs obtained from each condyle meet at an apex which is the most retruded position. If patients find difficulty in achieving the retruded position this will be seen on the tracing where both the arcs meet

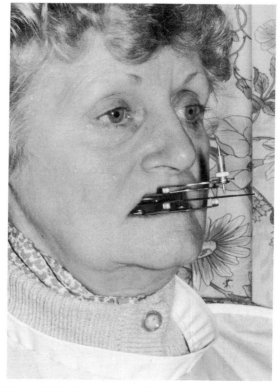

Figure 5.8 Gothic arch tracing device

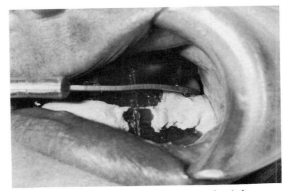

Figure 5.10 Facebow fork fitted to upper occlusal rim

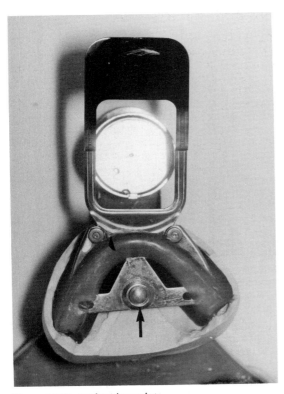

Figure 5.9 Centre bearing point

in a rounded curve rather than in a sharp point. By practice, however, and the fact that the patient finds no obstruction to lateral movement soon allows the retruded position to be achieved. It can then be recorded as before by placing a rapid setting material between the rims.

The facebow record

The use of a facebow to accurately position the cast in the articulator is an essential procedure if the occlusion of the natural teeth is to be examined or restored but where, as in complete dentures, the bases rest on a movable foundation capable of considerable displacement a doubt exists as to its necessity. It can be demonstrated that failure to use the facebow in complete denture construction and given the greatest possible error in placing the cast in the articulator, the intercuspal error is small in comparison with the amount of denture displacement. For this reason therefore facebows are not always used. However, if it is decided that a facebow record is necessary the procedure is similar to that described in Chapter 2 and following the recording of the centric jaw relationship, the occlusal fork is

embedded in the upper wax rim ensuring that the record is not damaged and (Figure 5.10) that the centre lines, canine lines and lip lines are not obliterated. The records are placed back in the patient's mouth and with the patient holding the rims together the facebow is positioned. In order to set the condyle mechanism to that of the patient and also to take into account the Bennett movement, protrusive and lateral jaw records should be taken. With complete dentures it is important that a centre bearing point be used as any attempt to obtain other than centric records will cause the bases to be displaced or compression of the underlying tissues to take place. For this reason, taking the centric and eccentric records together with a facebow at the same time can create difficulties and separate patient visits are advisable. The trial stage is an ideal time to do this as the denture can be set up to an average condyle angle of 30° and the adjustments made immediately before processing the denture. The technique of obtaining the eccentric records will be discussed at the trial stage.

Selection of teeth

The anterior artificial teeth are made in different shapes, sizes and colours and different materials. The posterior teeth, in addition to these factors, also have different occlusal forms. Before the records and facebow are sent to the laboratory the anterior and posterior teeth must be selected.

Selection of mould (shape) (Figure 5.11)

All guides for artificial teeth are arranged in square, tapering and ovoid forms following the Leon Williams classification. It was argued that the shape of the upper central incisor teeth is the same shape as the face inverted. There is little scientific

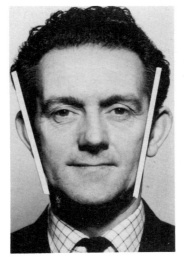
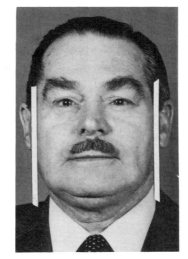
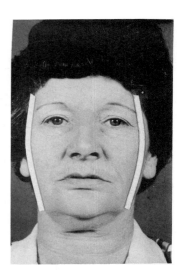

Figure 5.11 Selection of the tooth shape

evidence to show that this is in fact correct. Lee (1962) has described a method of tooth selection in which three facial measurements were selected to give the proportions of the teeth to the proportions of the face: (i) the width of the front of the forehead, (ii) the width of the front of the face at the level of the lips and (iii) width of the face across the zygoma. This should correspond to the dimensions of the gingival third, incisal tip and the maximum tooth width.

The size

The size of the teeth will depend on the amount of space available and this can be assessed from the occlusal rim. In order to obtain the length of the tooth and the actual width of the tooth a flexible ruler is used to measure the distance between the canine lines on the occlusal rim (Figure 5.12). Most mould guides give the width of the upper six anterior teeth and dividers can be used to measure the intercanine width on a set of teeth usually contained in a selection of moulds (Figure 5.13) and compared with the measurement from the occlusal rim. Widths of six anterior teeth arranged on an arc are generally about 3 mm wider than the width of the nose (the intercanine width).

Selection of shade

Artificial teeth are supplied with different shade guides and the selection of the ideal colour for the patient will depend upon the patient's own wishes but should depend also on the age of the patient, the colour of the skin and be selected to give a harmonious result. Patients with advancing years would be expected to have darker teeth than young patients.

Selection of material

Artificial teeth are generally made in either porcelain, which has a hard glazed surface or in acrylic resins. Porcelain is not easily abraded by cleaning agents or food and is not affected by solvents and thus the long-term aesthetics of anterior porcelain teeth are extremely good whilst acrylic teeth on the other hand may become worn with consequent loss of appearance. Likewise, posterior teeth in acrylic resin tend to wear with loss of the vertical dimension but porcelain posterior

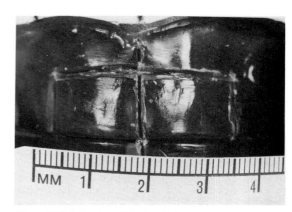

Figure 5.12 Selection of the tooth size

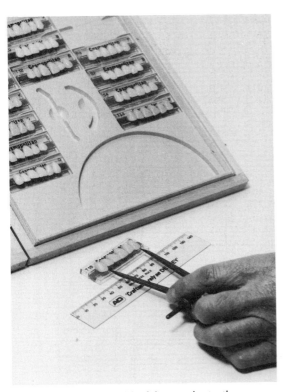

Figure 5.13 Selecting width of the anterior teeth

teeth can also chip and break under masticatory force and patients often do not like the sound of the porcelain teeth as they come into contact. Acrylic resin teeth have the advantage also that they bond to the denture base by chemical union whilst porcelain teeth must be held by mechanical means. The present extensive use of acrylic resin teeth has, on economic grounds, led to a situation where few patients are prepared to accept porcelain teeth although they are in the main preferable.

Completion of the work card

The necessary details of the size, shape, etc., concerning the teeth selected are now entered on the patient's work card and the clinical records are placed in an antiseptic solution and the facebow washed prior to being transferred to the laboratory (Figure 5.14).

Aesthetics

Aesthetics is the art of relating the teeth to the face to produce an overall pleasurable result. This thus involves the selection of the teeth in size, shape, colour and material as well as the arrangement. The arrangement will change with each person varying the amount of tooth seen together with the angulation, etc. This is a study in itself and is of an artistic nature and reference should be made to a number of texts on this subject.

CLINICIAN:

TECHNICIAN:

TYPE OF WORK: CD/ -/CD P/ /P OVERDENTURE

Obturator

Immediate

Technical instructions

_____

_____

_____

_____

_____

_____

_____

_____

_____

_____

_____

_____

_____

_____

_____

_____

_____

Staff Sig.	Student	Clinical stage	Next appointment
		Primary Impression	
		Final Impression	
		Jaw relation record	
		Wax trial 1	
		Wax trial 2	
		Metal trial	
		Insert denture	
		Review	

Shade	Mould	Posteriors	
		Anatomical/Cuspless	
Special tray material		Design approved:	
Articulator			

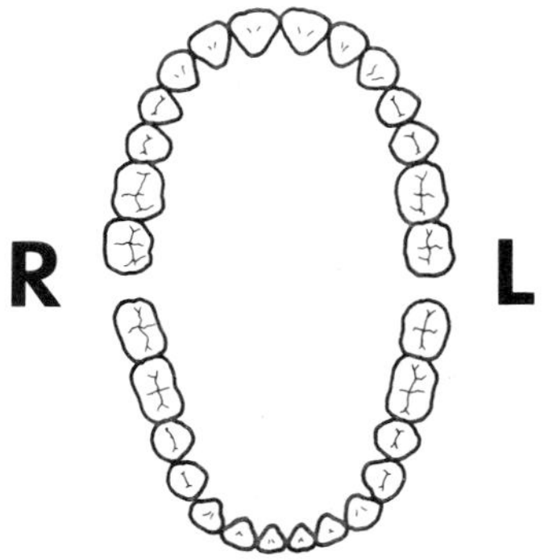

R   L

Figure 5.14 A work card

6

Mounting casts on an articulator

It is an advantage in many instances to remount appliances after processing whilst still on the master casts. The split mounting procedure facilitates the remounting of casts and dentures on an articulator after processing. To effect this cast mounting procedure, the base of the cast must be modified. Either the periphery of the base is chamferred and grooves are cut at right angles to each other or, alternatively, the base may be notched (Figure 6.1). After the base has been prepared, a sodium alginate separating medium is applied over the base to permit detachment of the cast from the articulator mounting plaster (Figure 6.2). Small undercuts may be cut in the sides of the cast to prevent the mounting plaster and cast separating prematurely.

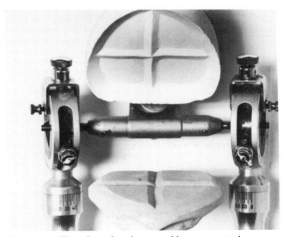

Figure 6.2 Chamferred and grooved base mounted on articulator

It is, however, possible to purchase special plates for this purpose (Figure 6.3). The plates are in two parts, held together with a large pin and, during use, one half is held in the mounting plaster and the other half in the base of the cast. To remove the cast from the articulator, the pin is removed and the two plates separated.

Complete dentures

There are a large number of articulators available, but the most complicated, such as the Denar (Figure 6.4), are seldom used for complete denture construction. They are more widely used for fixed restorations. The Dentatus articulator is, however,

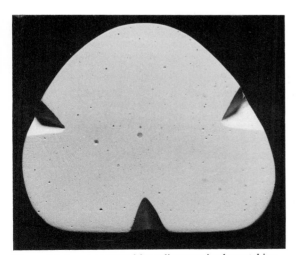

Figure 6.1 A cast prepared for split mounting by notching the periphery

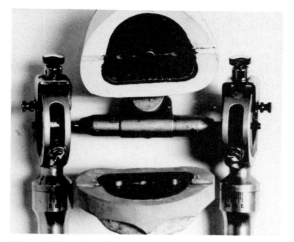

Figure 6.3 Special split cast mounting plates

capable of reproducing jaw movements when properly adjusted to fine limits and is more than adequate for most removable denture constructions.

Dentatus articulator

The following technique describes the procedure for mounting the master casts on a Dentatus articulator (Figure 6.5a), but there are also a large number of other articulators of a similar type (Hanau), to which this same description would apply. The first and foremost step is to prepare the cast for split mounting; the articulator is locked with the condylar ball in its central position, so the upper arm will then only rotate as a hinge. It is essential to ensure that the locking screw which allows for retrusive movements of the jaw (forward movements of the upper arm of the articulator) is screwed into its fullest depth. The incisal guidance pin should be set at zero, with the upper arm of the articulator parallel to the lower arm. The incisal guidance table must be set horizontal. The facebow is now positioned on the articulator, but it is generally found that the articulator is narrower than the patient's face. It is therefore necessary to adjust the condyle rods (Figure 6.5aA). It is essential that the two rods be moved in equal amounts in order to maintain the same centre line on the articulator as on the patient. In some articulators, instead of altering the facebow, the condylar mechanisms have small rods which are extended to meet the sliding rods of the facebow. These are adjusted to be equal on both sides (Figure 6.5c). The height is adjusted by the screw to allow the infra-orbital pointer to touch the infra-orbital plate (Figure 6.5aD). The upper cast is placed in the occlusal rim (Figure 6.6) and the cast will then be positioned in the same

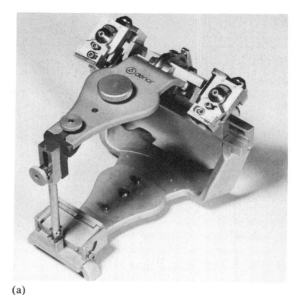

(a)

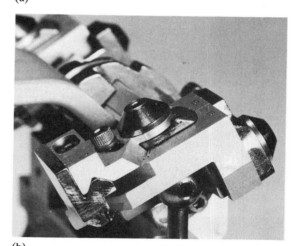

(b)

Figure 6.4 The Denar articulator (a) and the condylar mechanism (b)

relationship on the articulator to the condylar mechanism as the maxilla is to the temporomandibular joint when the Frankfurt plane of the patient is horizontal. The cast is then covered in a layer of mixed plaster of Paris and the upper arm is lowered so that the incisal guidance pin touches the incisal guidance table.

When the attaching plaster has reached a preliminary set, it is carved to the final shape (Figure 6.7), the facebow fork is removed from the upper occlusal rim, being careful not to damage the recording. The articulator is turned upside down and the lower occlusal rim placed into position on the upper and the lower cast seated in the occlusal

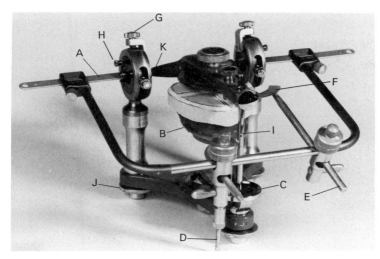

Figure 6.5(a) The Dentatus articulator with the upper cast supported by means of a facebow. A, condyle rods; B, facebow fork; C, incisal guidance table; D, height adjusting screw; E, infra-orbital pointer; F, frankfurt plane indicator; G, locking mechanism for fixing slope of 'condyle'; H, locking mechanism for the 'condyle ball'; J, locking mechanism for pillar rotation to allow for Bennett movement; K, mechanism allowing the 'condyle' to move forwards, downwards, and inwards; L, incisal guidance pin

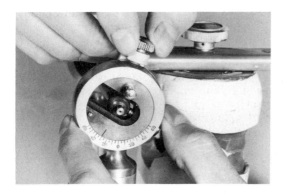

Figure 6.5(b) Adjusting the condylar slope

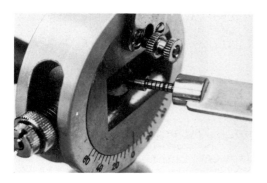

Figure 6.5(c) The 'condyle' mechanism of the articulator adjusted to meet the facebow rods as an alternative to moving the latter to fit the articulator

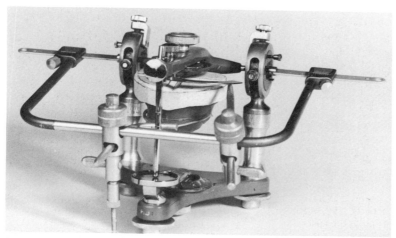

Figure 6.6 An upper edentulous cast placed in the occlusal rim prior to plastering to the articulator

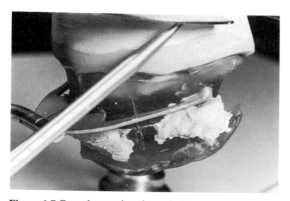

Figure 6.7 Cast plastered to the articulator

rim. The assembled casts must be held firmly together with rods and sticky wax, or an elastic band passing around the casts, and a further mix of plaster is placed on the base of the lower cast. The articulator is closed so that the plaster enters the mounting ring as in the attachment of the upper cast (Figure 6.8) . When the plaster has finally set, this is smoothed and the articulator is then ready for the setting up of the teeth in the occlusal rims.

If a Dentatus articulator is being used, but without the facebow, casts are placed in the occlusal rims and sealed in position. A mound of Plasticine is placed on the lower mounting plate and the assembled casts lowered onto it with the occlusal plane of the upper occlusal rim parallel to the lower arm and level with the incisal mark on the incisal guidance pin (Figure 6.9). Plaster is placed on the

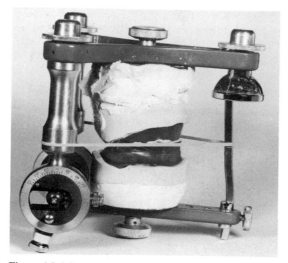

Figure 6.8 A lower cast being attached to the mounting plate

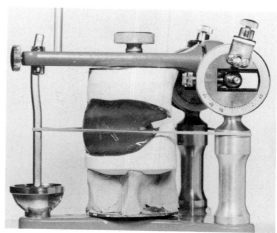

Figure 6.9 Mounting edentulous cast with the aid of occlusal rims in the articulator without the use of a facebow

base of the upper cast and the upper arm is lowered. Care must be taken to ensure that there is sufficient space between the mounting plate and the cast, so that the incisal guidance pin can touch the table. When set, the plaster is trimmed and smoothed in exactly the same way as described earlier. The articulator is then inverted and the lower cast attached as above.

Average condylar path articulators

Some articulators (e.g. Freeplane 75 and Gysi simplex) are supplied with occlusal mounting tables. This provides a plane of orientation in the articulator which facilitates the mounting of the cast. In addition, the occlusal plane table simplifies the arrangement of the teeth and this will be described in Chapter 7.

The casts are prepared as previously described for the split cast technique. The upper occlusal rim is placed centrally on the mounting table, and if a centre line is available it should be used. The upper cast is placed in the occlusal rim, plaster is placed on the base of the cast and the upper arm is lowered into it, as decribed previously (Figure 6.10). When the plaster has reached a preliminary set, the mounting table may be removed and the lower cast and occlusal rim secured to the upper with rods and sticky wax or by an elastic band. Plaster is then added to the lower arm of the articulator and the cast lowered onto it. The plaster is trimmed and smoothed and the articulator is then ready for the setting up of the teeth (Figure 6.11).

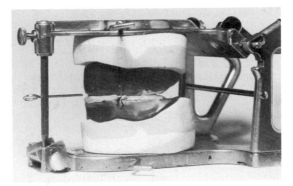

Figure 6.11 The casts mounted in the articulator

If no mounting table is available, the procedure is exactly the same as that described for the Dentatus articulator without the facebow.

Cast mounting on a hinge

Occasionally, and this will become clear in Chapter 7, the use of a hinge to approximate the casts may be all that is required. The rims are secured to the casts and held together by rods, sticky wax or an elastic band (as previously described). The mix of plaster of Paris is made and placed around the lower arm of the hinge. The lower cast is then lowered onto the plaster, ensuring that the occlusal plane is parallel to the bench and that the arms of the hinge are centrally placed along the mid-line of the upper. More plaster is added to the upper cast and the upper arm lowered into and covered by it. When set, the plaster is trimmed and smoothed and the adjustable screw set to the vertical dimension and the locking nut tightened (Figure 6.12). Divider recordings of the vertical dimension should also be registered on the sides of the cast, to allow for any movement of the locking screw (see Figure 7.4).

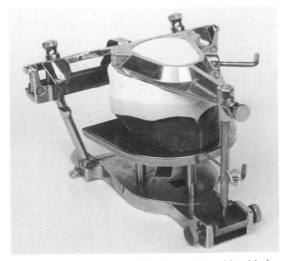

Figure 6.10 The Freeplane 75 and mounting table with the occlusal rim and upper cast plastered to the articulator

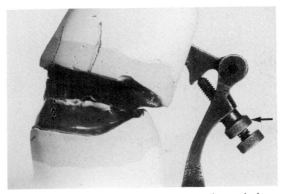

Figure 6.12 Hinge locking nut set to correct the vertical dimension

Mounting dentate casts

The procedure for mounting diagnostic or master casts is exactly the same. It must be remembered, however, that mounting diagnostic casts may not be necessary if, on examination of the patient clinically, the occlusion is satisfactory, or if so many teeth have been lost that no occlusion posteriorly exists and only the anterior teeth are standing, or when one jaw is edentulous. Also, if only some posterior teeth are present, it may not be possible to use an interocclusal record and occlusal rims will be required to obtain an accurate record of the relationship of the lower jaw to the maxilla. The facebow is positioned on the articulator, which must be an adjustable one, such as a Dentatus, which has previously been locked and set as described on page 36. The split cast technique is not used when mounting dentate casts. The upper cast is placed in the facebow fork and the screw is adjusted to raise the infra-orbital pointer, if used, to the infra-orbital plate. The plaster mix is then placed on top of the cast and the upper bow is lowered until the plaster

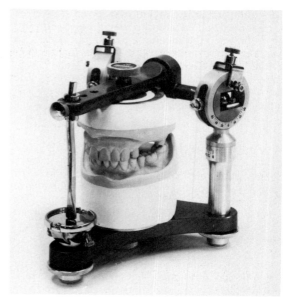

Figure 6.14 Dentate casts mounted in a Dentatus articulator

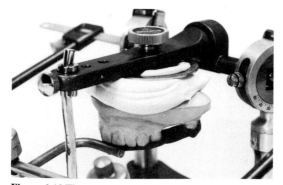

Figure 6.13 The upper cast mounted with the facebow

flows into the mounting ring (Figure 6.13). When the plaster has reached its initial set the facebow is removed. The plaster is smoothed and the articulator turned over. The two casts are approximated using a centric interocclusal record and a mix of plaster placed on the base of the lower cast. A similar procedure is then used to attach the lower cast to the lower mounting ring. When finally set, the plaster is smoothed and the study casts are ready to be examined. The centric interocclusal record is removed and the casts approximated. The teeth should be in centric occlusion (Figure 6.14).

7

Setting up artificial teeth for complete dentures

Having mounted the occlusal rims in the articulator, setting up the artificial teeth can be started, but, before doing so, adjustment of the articulator may be necessary.

There are five factors in the laws of occlusion as originally stated by Hanau (Hickey, Zarb and Bolender, 1985). They are condylar guidance angle, the incisal guidance angle, cuspal angle, orientation of the occlusal plane and the prominence of the compensating curve. The incisal guidance and the condylar guidance angles are factors which are set on the articulator and the remainder are related to the arrangement of the teeth. In both the Dentatus and the free plane 75, the incisal guidance must be set as this controls the vertical and horizontal overlap of the teeth. If cuspless teeth are used, special conditions exist which will be discussed later. The vertical overlap (overbite) may be defined as the distance the maxillary teeth extend over the mandibular teeth in a vertical direction (Figure 7.1) and the horizontal overlap (overjet) is the distance the maxillary teeth project beyond the mandibular teeth in the horizontal direction. For most patients when using anatomical posterior teeth, the incisal guidance table is set at 10°; thus allowing enough overlap to give reasonable aesthetics and, at the same time, have a minimum of influence on the setting up of the teeth. The condylar guidance for the Dentatus may be individually adjusted by using interocclusal records, or may be set to an average value. The individual adjustment of the articulator, using interocclusal records, is described at the trial stage of the denture, but, for setting the teeth, the condylar guidance is arranged as an average value, which is usually 30° to the horizontal. The Bennett movement is controlled by the vertical rotation of the pillars supporting the condylar mechanism and these are set using a formula H/8 + 12. For example,

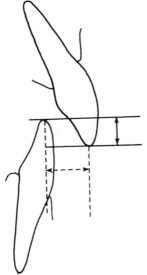

Figure 7.1 The vertical and horizontal overlap of the anterior teeth

if the condylar inclination is 30° on each side, the lateral inclination setting is 30°/8 + 12 = 16°. This setting is made by adjusting the horizontal vernier scale shown in Figure 7.2. When individual interocclusal records are used the lateral records will determine the Bennett movement and the rotation of the pillars will be made for each individual.

The two settings, i.e. the incisal guidance and condylar guidance, control the movement of the articulator and establish a rotation centre, shown in Figure 7.3a for protrusive movement and Figure 7.3b for lateral movements.

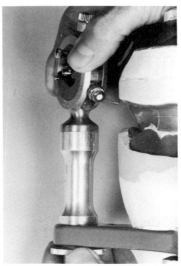

Figure 7.2 Adjustment of the Bennett movement by rotation of the vertical pillars

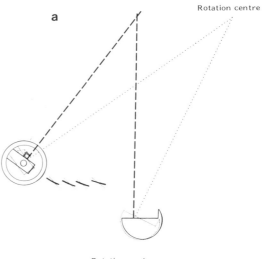

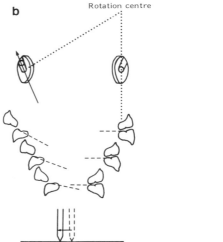

Figure 7.3 (a) The rotation centre created by the condyler angle and the incisal guidance for protrusive movements, and (b) the rotation centre for lateral movements. The centre will move from side to side depending on which lateral movement is carried out

The cusps of the artificial teeth must therefore lie on arcs from this centre if balanced articulation is to be achieved. It can be seen that if the condylar angle changes the steepness of the arc will also change. This will occur also if the incisal guidance table is altered, since the rotation centre will be changed. When setting shallow cusp teeth, therefore, the compensating curve will have to be increased and vice versa. The occlusal plane is controlled by clinical conditions and is established with the occlusal rims and it is therefore unwise to change this in the laboratory. Now that the articulator has been set to the required angles, the setting of the teeth can begin. In addition to centric jaw relationship, the upper rim will have been trimmed and contoured to give the correct lip support and also the occlusal rims prescribe to the technician the details of the buccolingual tooth position. The incisal edge level, occlusal plane level, centre line, the canine position (cusp point) and the high smile line will also have been marked on the rims.

As the teeth are set into the occlusal rim, this recorded information is destroyed. Thus, it is essential to transfer these data onto the articulator mounting plaster so that checks on tooth positioning may be made. Reference to Figure 7.4 shows the centre line scribed onto the mounting plaster. Using a pair of dividers set at an arbitrary opening, the incisal edge level and the high smile line can also be scribed onto the plaster. The divider setting is scribed onto the side or base of the plaster mounting as a reference.

As the upper rim has been trimmed to give the occlusal plane level, the lower rim should be restored to occlude with the upper rim to facilitate an occlusal plane guide for setting the upper teeth.

Alternatively, a flat metal plate or occlusal plane table may be used.

The make and shade of teeth required, the upper anterior mould size and type of posterior tooth form will have been selected and prescribed by the clinician.

The size of the lower anteriors is dependent on the upper mould size and the tooth manufacturer's mould guide chart will indicate the appropriate size for Class I relationships. In a Class II anterior tooth relationship, because of the retruded and narrow arch form, it is necessary to select a smaller mould. Conversely, in a Class III relationship, a larger mould of lower tooth or an additional incisor tooth

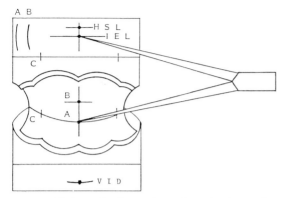

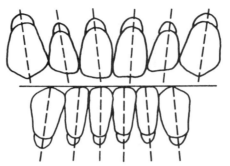

Figure 7.5 The arrangement of the anterior teeth

Figure 7.4 Information is transferred from the rims to the mounting plaster by the use of dividers and marking knife. The centre line, canine line (C), high smile line (HSL), incisal edge level (IEL) and the vertical inter-cast dimension (VID) are marked. The divider settings must be recorded (A, B)

may be used. These relationships are discussed later in this chapter.

Tooth positioning

There are a variety of techniques and procedures that may be employed in 'setting up' that will give the desired result, but the one described here has proved to be one of the easiest to understand and carry out. Regardless of the articulator used, the upper anterior teeth are set first. They are set within the wax contoured occlusal rim and must be confined within the labial contour which has been trimmed to give the required lip support.

Setting up anterior teeth

The classic arrangement of the upper six anteriors is shown in Figure 7.5. First, an upper central incisor is positioned. This ensures correct establishment of the midline position. With the centrals, the long axis should be slightly inclined to the vertical when seen from the front and inclined downwards and slightly forwards when seen from the side at an angle of 108° to the Frankfurt plane. The incisal edge should lie on the occlusal plane (Figure 7.6).

The lateral incisor is set next. It is inclined with the neck positioned more distally than the incisal edges and the neck set in more than the central. The incisal edge should be parallel to the occlusal plane, but about 1 mm above (Figure 7.7).

The canine is set with its long axis towards the centre line. The centre of the incisal edge (the cusp point) should contact the occlusal plane. The approximal long axes are vertical, which produces a slight prominence of the neck of these teeth. The

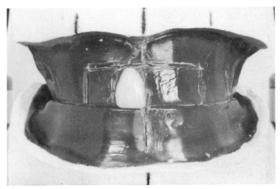

Figure 7.6 The position of the central incisor on the occlusal plane

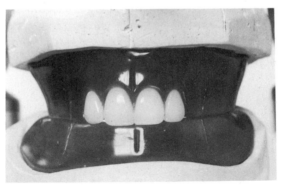

Figure 7.7 The lateral incisors 1 mm above and parallel to the occlusal plane

central, lateral and canine of the opposite side are then set (Figure 7.8).

Some technicians prefer to lay down a new base plate and set the teeth upon it, thus keeping the centric jaw record as a reference, but this presents certain difficulties in getting the teeth in their correct position with respect to the lips and the neutral zone. If such a technique is used, a piece of softened wax is placed on the base and the tooth positioned correctly and then molten wax is flowed, with a wax knife, around the tooth to form a

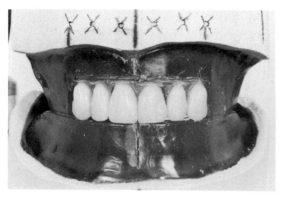

Figure 7.8 The six anteriors are now in position

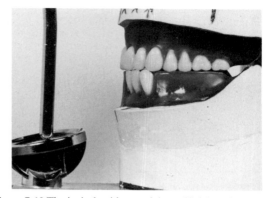

Figure 7.10 The incisal guidance of the artificial teeth

gingivae. With this method the scribed marks on the mounting plaster and the use of dividers are essential to obtain the correct height and position of the teeth.

A better method is to remove a piece of wax from the occlusal rim, in the region of the tooth to be positioned and, using a hot wax knife, softening the rim prior to placing the tooth in position. Place an upper central first to obtain the correct centre line, followed by the lateral and canine teeth as described earlier. Wax is again flowed around the teeth and smoothed to form the lost alveolus and the gingivae.

The setting order is the same for the lower teeth. The long axis inclinations of these teeth is shown in Figure 7.5 and Figure 7.9. The lower anteriors are

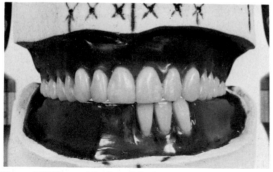

Figure 7.9 The positioning of the lower anterior teeth

set in exactly the same way as the upper teeth and positioned to give a 1 mm vertical overlap and a 1 mm horizontal one in relation to the upper teeth. This amounts to a low incisal guidance of about 10° (Figure 7.10) and when the incisal guidance pin is moved on the plate, balance should be established in protrusive and lateral movements. The lower anteriors may need painstaking and meticulous adjustment to establish this balance and variations in horizontal and vertical overlap may be required as a consequence of the patient's aesthetic or phonetic needs.

Setting up the maxillary posterior teeth

The major consideration in setting up posterior teeth is that the maxillary teeth must be so arranged that they will remain in correct relationship to the opposing mandibular teeth, not only in centric occlusion, but also during lateral and protrusive movements of the mandible. The cusps of these teeth must therefore lie on arcs from the rotation centre.

The first procedure is to mark the crest of the lower ridge with a pencil from the retromolar pad through the canine area on both sides of the cast. Using a straight edge, the line is extended both anteriorly and posteriorly onto the land of the cast (Figure 7.11). The lower rim is then placed onto the cast and, using the straight edge, a line is scribed on the occlusal surface of the rim to correspond with the pencil line on the cast (Figure 7.12). This line is used to align the palatal cusps of the upper posterior teeth. The plane of occlusion of the posterior teeth is obtained from the level of the lower occlusal rim and the first procedure is to remove a piece of wax from the occlusal rim and soften the remaining wax and place the upper left first premolar (bicuspid).

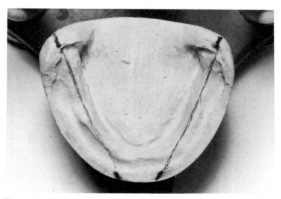

Figure 7.11 The cast marked to indicate the lower ridge

When in position correctly both its cusps should touch the plane of occlusion (represented by the lower rim) and its long axis should be at right angles to the plane with the palatal cusp over the crest of

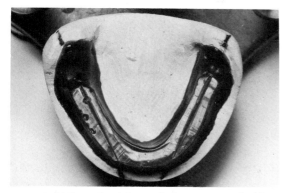

Figure 7.12 The occlusal rim marked to correspond with the line on the cast

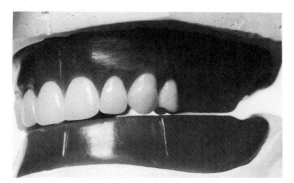

Figure 7.13 The upper first premolar (bicuspid) placed with cusps on the occlusal plane and the lingual cusp on the ridge line

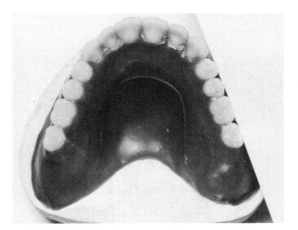

Figure 7.14 Labial surface of the canine and the bicuspids in a straight line

the lower ridge, i.e. on the line scribed onto the lower rim (Figure 7.13). The upper second premolar (bicuspid) is then set in the same way. The buccal surfaces of the premolars (bicuspids) and the labial surfaces of the canine should be in line (Figure 7.14). The molar teeth have shallower cusps than the premolars (bicuspids) and, in order to achieve balance, it is necessary to tilt the teeth so that they will lie on the arcs from the rotation centre. This tilting of the tooth produces curved planes of occlusion, which are commonly called the compensating curves, one anteroposteriorly and one laterally. In order to achieve this, the maxillary first molar is set in the wax with its mesial lingual cusp on the plane of occlusion and over the crest of the lower ridge and on the scribed line, whilst the mesiobuccal and distobuccal and distolingual cusps should be raised approximately 0.75 mm from the plane. This, thus, starts the compensating curves. The second molar is then placed with its cusps from between 0.75–1.00 mm above the plane of occlusion (Figure 7.15). The same procedure is used to set the posteriors on the opposite side (Figure 7.16).

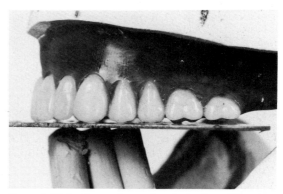

Figure 7.15 The first and second molar teeth positioned to create the compensating curve

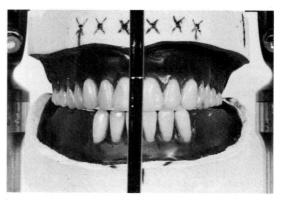

Figure 7.16 The set-up of the maxillary posterior teeth completed

Arranging the mandibular posterior teeth

A piece of wax is removed from the area of the lower left second premolar (bicuspid) and the tooth position over the crest of the lower ridge. The buccal cusp should occlude between the maxillary first and second premolars and contact their marginal ridges and its lingual cusp should fit between the lingual cusp of the two maxillary bicuspids or premolars. This places the mandibular second premolar in centric occlusion.

If the articulator is now released and the upper arm of the articulator moved to the patient's right, the buccal cusp of the upper first premolar should be in contact with the buccal cusp of the lower second premolar thus establishing a working contact (Figure 7.17). Similarly, if the articulator is released

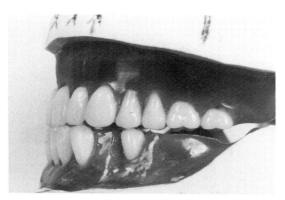

Figure 7.17 The establishment of the balancing contact between the palatal cusp of the upper first premolar with the buccal cusp of the lower second premolar

and the upper arm moved to the patient's left, i.e. the operator's right facing the set-up, the buccal cusp of the mandibular second premolar should contact the lingual cusp of the maxillary first premolar (Figure 7.18).

The next tooth to be positioned is the lower left first molar tooth. This is positioned such that the mesiobuccal cusp will occlude with the marginal ridges of the upper second premolar and the upper first molar, whilst the distobuccal cusp will occlude with the central fossa of the upper first molar. The mesiolingual cusp of the upper first molar should be well seated into the central fossa of the lower tooth, if the condylar mechanism is then released, working, balancing and protrusive postions of the tooth can be established and any necessary adjustments made. No interference should occur whilst translating from one position to another and the incisal guidance pin should remain on the incisal guidance table throughout. A tight centric occlusion should be re-verified

and the balancing articulation checked again before wax is added around the tooth to form the necessary alveolar and gum tissue (Figure 7.19).

The first premolar is now positioned. Depending on the jaw relationship, the space for this tooth may be variable and in those patients with a retrusive jaw

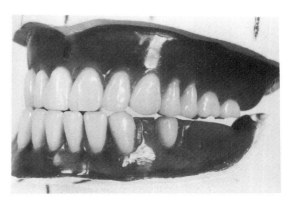

Figure 7.18 Balancing contact achieved between the buccal cusp of the mandibular second premolar and the palatal cusp of the maxillary first premolar

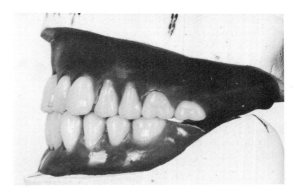

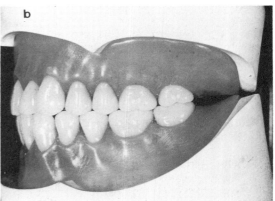

Figure 7.19 Central occlusion verified (a) and wax added (b) to form gum work

(Class II) inadequate space may exist when the tooth will have to be ground in its mesiodistal width to be able to be positioned. Likewise, in Class III situations, where the lower jaw is larger than the upper, the space may be somewhat larger and a wider tooth may be necessary.

In normal jaws, the first premolar is positioned so that its buccal cusp is between the maxillary premolar and the canine tooth in centric relation (Figure 7.20). When the articulator is moved into a

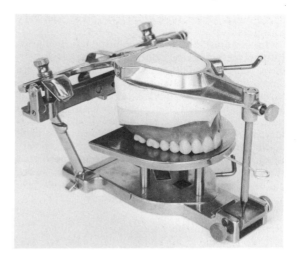

Figure 7.21 Plane guide table being used to assist in the development of the compensating curve when setting the maxillary bicuspids and molar teeth

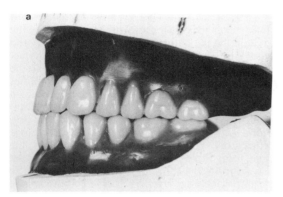

Figure 7.20 Contact between the buccal cusp of the mandibular first premolar and the distal incisal edge of the maxillary canine and mesial occlusal edge of the maxillary first premolar takes place when in a working occlusion

working occlusion the tooth should lie with the buccal cusp in contact with the distoincisal edge of the maxillary canine and the mesioocclusal edge of the buccal cusp of the maxillary first premolar. In the balancing situation, the first premolar tooth is completely free and has no balancing function.

The second molar is dealt with in exactly the same manner, establishing centric occlusion with the mesiobuccal cusp being positioned between and on the marginal ridges of the first upper and second molars. The distobuccal cusp fits into the central fossa of the upper second molar and the mesio-palatal cusp of the second upper molar fits into the central fossa of the lower second molar. Balancing, working and protrusive contact are established in exactly the same way as for the first molar.

Setting up teeth using the average value articulator

Generally, average value articulators have adjustable incisal guidance tables, but non-adjustable condylar elements which are usually set at 30°. Most average value articulators are also supplied with plane guide tables which assist in the setting-up procedures (Figure 7.21). One procedure, which is a variation on that previously described using an adjustable articulator, is as follows.

Having restored the lower rim, the ridge crest line is scribed as described earlier and the upper rim trimmed to correspond with this line. It thus enables the upper tooth to be positioned correctly in relation to the lower ridge. With the occlusal plane table in place and the upper anteriors set as previously described, the upper posterior teeth are set in a similar manner, using the guide table to establish the compensating curve. It will be appreciated that the lingual cusp of the upper posteriors, if set on the line which represents the crest of the lower ridge (which is indicated by the pre-trimmed upper rim), will ensure that the lower posteriors are set over the crest of the ridge. In most cases this will be the position to offer maximum stability. Once the upper posteriors are set the table is removed and the lower occlusal rim placed in position. This is reduced as necessary and the teeth are positioned in exactly the same way as previously described, starting with the lower anteriors and then proceeding with the posteriors.

Techniques for setting up cuspless teeth

There are may types of cuspless teeth and a variety of terms have been used to describe them, i.e. monoplane, inverted cusped, zero degree, non-anatomic, flat plane and several other terms which are usually related to a specific manufacturer's name. The flat occlusal surface is often the only factor they all have in common. Other factors such as depth of inverted cusp, crushing area, spillways, buccolingual width, type of material, cost, etc. vary considerably.

On an adjustable, or semi-adjustable articulator, cuspless teeth must still conform to the movement of the articulator and the teeth must lie on an arc from the rotation centre. In order to accommodate this curvature between the ridges of the cast, it is necessary to adjust the position of the rotation centre to be above the articulator. If the centre is forward of the articulator and a long way away from it, the steepness of the curve will necessitate very small lower anterior teeth and very poor aesthetics (Figure 7.22). To move the centre, the incisal guidance table on the articulator is adjusted to have a negative incisal guidance (Figure 7.23). The

anterior teeth will have a normal horizontal overlap, but a negative vertical one with a space of approx. 1 mm between the tips of the teeth when looked at anteriorly.

The setting of the teeth proceeds as before, with the upper and lower anteriors being set first and movement of the articulator ensuring balanced articulation of the anterior teeth in protrusion. The posteriors are set to an anteroposterior and lateral curve to obtain balance in all movements of the articulator. This curve will have its centre at the rotation centre of the articulator and is usually about 4 inches (10 cm). This is very similar to the curve of 4-inch radius which Monson (1922) proposed as the curvature of the natural teeth, when each cusp and incisal edge would touch this curve. Some manufacturers produce curved plates of this type to help the development of the occlusal plane which simplifies the setting of the teeth. It can be used for setting up cusped teeth, but the technique is not recommended. For cuspless teeth, however, it can be very helpful and can be used with a straight line hinge (articulator). When setting teeth on a straight line hinge, using these plates, the upper anteriors are set first according to the required lip support, centre line and incisal edge level. The curved occlusal plane guide is then positioned on a roll of Plasticine conformed to the lower cast (Figure 7.24). The plane is adjusted to orientate to the plane of occlusion which anteriorly is now determined by the upper anteriors. The upper cuspless posterior teeth

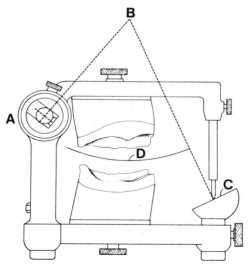

Figure 7.22 A set-up showing a steep curve with posterior cuspless teeth which necessitates very low and small anterior teeth

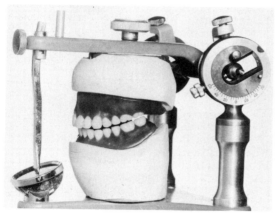

Figure 7.23 The improvement in aesthetics when a negative incisal guidance is used. A, Condylar guidance; B, rotation centre; C, incisal guidance; D, occlusal plane

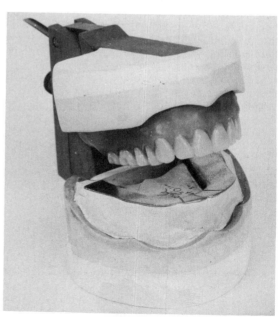

Figure 7.24 The curved occlusal plane guide is positioned on a roll of Plasticine placed over the lower ridge

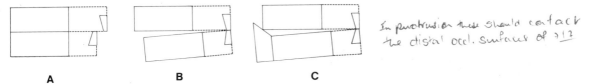

A   B   C

In protrusion these should contact the distal occl. surfaces of 7|7

Figure 7.25 The use of balancing ramps to compensate for the Christiansen effect. A, Centric occlusion; B, protrusion to show Christiansen effect; C, with balancing ramp

are then set with their occlusal surfaces fully contacting the plate. The Plasticine and plate are then removed and the lower teeth are set to the uppers. The level of the incisal edges of the lower anteriors must conform to the curved plate and therefore a negative incisal guidance will be achieved. This may be considered somewhat unaesthetic and, for this reason, the following method adopted by Sears (1949) is an advantage.

Three-point contact (Sears technique)

As an alternative to balanced articulation, three-point contact may be used. This is possible using balancing ramps to compensate for the Christiansen effect (Figure 7.25) and also provides zero incisal guidance for improved aesthetics. The occlusal rims are mounted in either an adjustable, semi-adjustable or straight line hinge articulator and the upper anteriors are set to the rim as previously described. The upper posteriors are set to a flat occlusal plane (Figure 7.26), the lower posteriors are set to occlude with the uppers and the incisal edges of the lower anteriors are set to the same plane level. In an adjustable or semi-adjustable articulator the lower second molar is tilted to produce contact in protrusion but in the straight line

hinge a mound of wax may be positioned distal to the lower molars at the clinical try-in stage (Figure 7.27) and the patient instructed to protrude to an edge-to-edge incisal relationship, thus recording the Christiansen effect (Figure 7.28). With this record, the variations of individual condylar path angulations are then allowed for in the set-up (Figure 7.29) by raising the second molar to the angle achieved on the wax.

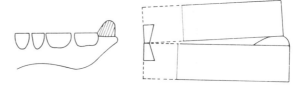

Figure 7.27 The use of a piece of wax to provide the level to which the distal contact should be produced to stabilize the denture by providing a posterior balancing ramp

Thus, a balancing ramp is produced in protrusion with one tooth in contact on the balancing side. In the working side movement, all the teeth on that side will be in contact (Figure 7.30).

A summary of the techniques used to obtain eccentric balance is shown in Table 7.1.

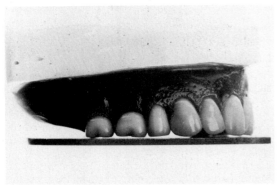

Figure 7.26 The setting-up of the flat occlusal plane with cuspless teeth shows a zero incisal guidance

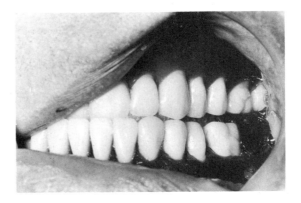

Figure 7.28 The protrusive record being produced

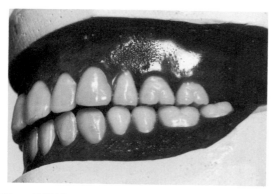

Figure 7.29 The second mandibular molar set to the established angle

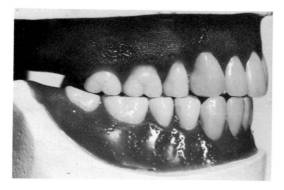

Figure 7.30 The balancing ramp operates on the balancing side only whilst on the working side the teeth are all in contact

Table 7.1 Eccentric balance

Cusp inclines in harmony with rotation centres determined by the condylar and incisal guidances

A Anatomical teeth and an adjustable articulator

B Cuspless teeth and a movable articulator
  (i) Negative incisal guidance
      Teeth set to protrusive and lateral curves determined by the articulator
  (ii) Zero incisal guidance
      Teeth set to a flat plane, balanced by tilting the last lower molar

C Cuspless teeth and a hinge articulator
  (i) Arbitrary curved templates
  (ii) Individual templates developed by the patient using plaster/pumice occlusal rims

Arrangement of posterior teeth in crossbite relationship

The relationship of the upper and lower ridges may present a situation where the maxillary arch is considerably narrower than the mandibular arch (Class III). In such cases, it is necessary to set the posteriors into what is commonly called a crossbite. Every effort should be made to avoid this by using a narrow (buccolingual) posterior tooth and placing it as lingually as possible, whilst bringing the upper posteriors as far buccally as is practical. However, variance between this technique and the use of a crossbite will need to be considered in each case, depending on the degree of severity of the crossbite relations. In cases where a crossbite is essential, the lower posteriors selected should be of a size larger than the uppers. This will facilitate the setting of the lower posteriors to the buccal of the uppers. Generally, the upper posteriors should be set with their buccal cusps over the crest of the lower ridge, rather than the lingual cusps as in the normal relationship (Figure 7.31). It has also been suggested that by crossing over the teeth, i.e. the upper left posterior teeth may be used for the right mandibular quadrant and the left lower for the right maxillary quadrant. This gives good articulation, although very poor aesthetics.

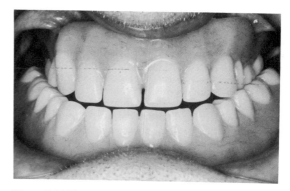

Figure 7.31 The arrangement of the posterior teeth in a cross-bite situation

Arrangement of the lower anteriors when the mandible is prominent is usually in what is termed an edge-to-edge relationship. The lower anteriors are set with their incisal edges in contact with the incisal edges of the upper anteriors. Wider lower anteriors may be selected to fill the space, or an extra incisor may be used.

Conversely, the lower arch may present a situation where it is considerably smaller than the upper arch (Class II). In such cases, a lower anterior tooth may be omitted, or a smaller mould of lower anteriors be used and, in setting up the posteriors, the first premolars (bicuspid) may be omitted, depending upon the amount of space available and the inter-arch relationships. It is not unusual to be faced with arch relationships that vary considerably from side to side. In such cases, it is important to achieve the optimum aesthetics and function without regard to symmetry.

Waxing up the trial dentures

The preparation of the trial denture involves shaping and contouring the polished surfaces of the dentures. The shape and contour will influence the fit, appearance, speech, comfort and retention. The waxed-up dentures should be of a form that is similar to the patient's natural soft tissues and harmonize with the oral facial musculature.

It is usual to wax up the upper denture first. The first and most important aspect of the upper denture is to ensure that the palate is of even thickness and this is probably best achieved when a base plate of shellac or autopolymerizing resin has been used. Trim back the surplus wax to the base plate, taking care not to disturb any teeth. Using a hot wax knife, flow wax over the necks of the teeth buccally, labially and palatally. Also add wax onto the flanges and overbuild the wax work slightly to allow for trimming and shaping. Build up the wax work in the lower denture in a similar fashion and then allow the wax to harden. When hard, the teeth are trimmed using a carver (Figure 7.32) fully exposing each tooth and ensuring that the gingival contours are at the height of the natural gingivae. These vary considerably at all ages and, in the elderly, some root will also be exposed. The interdental papillae should be pronounced and a close study of stone casts from a patient's natural teeth is recommended to ensure a lifelike appearance (Figure 7.33).

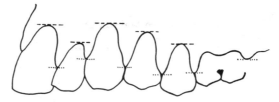

Figure 7.33 Note varying heights of the papillae. (From Frush and Fisher, 1958)

Likewise, the posterior teeth should be exposed and contoured. That part of the base, which represents the lost alveolar tissue, must now be shaped and contoured and, in the upper anteriors, the object is to create shallow root eminences with the canines having the greatest eminence (Figure 7.34). The laterals are smallest and the centrals should fall between the two. The buccal surfaces require little or no contouring. With these surfaces it is important that they should be carved to face downwards and outwards to aid retention. The palatal surface will face inwards and downwards. This is best understood by reference to Figure 7.35. The labial surface of the lower should be slightly concave, with the root eminences shallow or non-existent. A concavity on this surface allows for the contraction of the orbicularis oris to work as a seating force during function. The buccal surfaces of the lower require to be shaped so that they face outwards and upwards and thus aid retention. The lingual surfaces must be shaped to face inwards and upwards. The tongue should thus be able to stabilize the lower denture by acting as a seating force.

The natural gingivae have a slightly stippled appearance and some patients prefer their dentures to be the same. However, these small indentations can be the site of staining and, if it is used, it is preferable only in the upper denture in the anterior

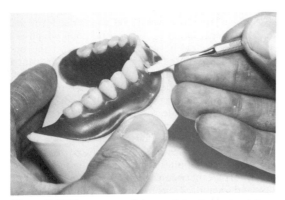

Figure 7.32 The wax round the teeth is trimmed to fully expose the tooth

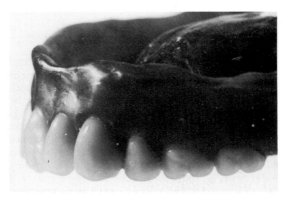

Figure 7.34 A set-up demonstrating the different root eminences to give a natural appearance

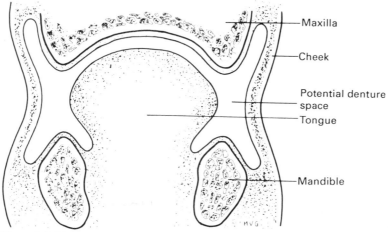

Figure 7.35 The shape of the palatal and buccal surface shapes. (From Beresin and Schiesser, 1973)

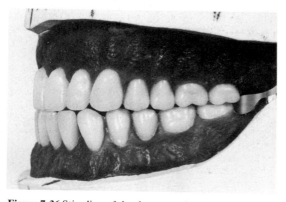

Figure 7.36 Stippling of the denture using a small stiff brush

region. This stippling may be achieved by using a small stiff brush (Figure 7.36).

Finally, the wax work requires to be smoothed and polished. If stippling has been used, it needs only to be passed through a brush flame to smooth the edges of the stippling and the remainder may be smoothed by rubbing with a cloth or by burnishing. This is then followed again by a fine brush flame which will blend in the anatomic carving and smooth the wax. The waxed denture base can then be given a high shine with a piece of cotton wool and soapy water. Finally, the trial denture should be removed from the cast and the edges cleaned and smoothed. The trial denture should then be washed and is then ready for the clinician to try in the patient.

Clinical trial of complete denture

The set-up and the articulator are returned to the surgery and, as before, it is essential to wash the appliances thoroughly, in the sight of the patient, before inserting them in the oral cavity. Use of a disinfectant is not recommended at this stage, since the wax may be damaged.

The upper denture base is inserted and the retention confirmed. The position of the upper teeth is assessed for lip support and angulation. In those patients with a normal jaw relationship the labial face of the central incisors should be 108° to the Frankfurt plane and the lip at rest should just cover the tooth but this may vary with a number of factors such as length of the upper lip, age of the patient and previous jaw relationships.

The lower denture should now be inserted and the height of the lower teeth assessed in relation to the lower lip. They are usually on the same level and should be positioned in the neutral zone which is a theoretical 'space' between the tongue on the one side and the lip on the other. If either muscle groups exert pressure on the denture it will be displaced. This 'space' is best described as a zone of minimal conflict of muscle activity and although the term neutral zone is one used in orthodontics, the situation with respect to a denture is quite different from that of the natural teeth as the denture is immediately displaced by either muscle group. The same principle applies to the posterior teeth where they must lie between the tongue and the cheeks. The assessment of the posterior tooth position is a very important aspect of the trial of the denture. The height of the posterior teeth is such that the tongue should just be above the level of the lingual cusps of the posterior teeth and, in this way, the denture will be held in place by the tongue during functional movements.

The patient is asked to relax and the jaw closed to ascertain that the centric occlusion and centric jaw relationships coincide and this can further be perfected by asking the patient to tap the teeth lightly together very rapidly. During relaxation the patient should be aware of a space between the teeth.

Speech can also be used to assess the vertical dimension and tooth position. The 's' sound is a very useful guide to the vertical dimension which will be satisfactory if the teeth do not touch when the 's' sound is produced. Jaw position during the exercise produces the 'closest speaking space' but this is not the same as the freeway space. The assessment of the vertical dimension by these two techniques is a very useful guide to ensuring that the vertical dimension of the dentures is not excessive.

The speaking of the letters 'v' and 'f' is also a general guide to the position of the upper anterior teeth in relation to the lower lip. If the upper anterior tooth position is incorrect the patient will find it difficult to pronounce these fricatives.

Lastly, the aesthetics are considered and the patient is asked to comment so that alterations can be made. The size, shade, etc. and position of the teeth are examined and if the patient is satisfied the dentures are ready for processing.

Lateral and protrusive records

The centre bearing point is placed in the dentures (Figure 7.37) and the point raised to allow the patient to slide without tooth contact. Repeated movements are practised to right and left lateral positions and also the protrusive position, and once the patient can undertake these movements and hold it for a minute, the records can be taken using a quick setting material. The best material is one which can be cleaned away easily from the teeth and will not damage the set-up. A polyether material is ideal for this purpose but silicone products are also available. The material is placed over the lower posterior teeth and the patient's jaw guided into one of the eccentric positions (Figure 7.38). It is held there until the material is set and the material can then be removed and the remaining records taken. Each record must be recorded carefully as it will be returned, with the articulator and the set-up, to the laboratory for the final adjustment prior to finishing.

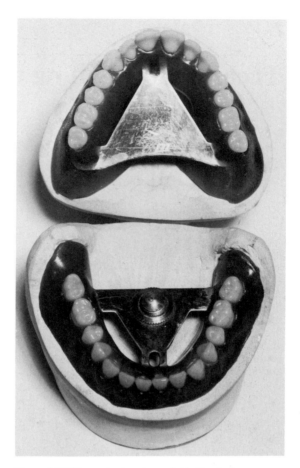

Figure 7.37 The centre bearing point in the dentures allowing the patient to slide from side to side without tooth contact

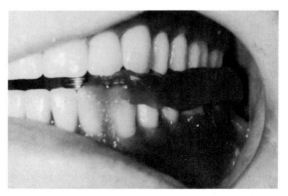

Figure 7.38 The eccentric jaw records being produced using a wax material

Treatment planning and partial dentures

Having examined the patient and assembled all the data as described in Chapter 1 a sequential plan of the treatment is necessary. This is essential for two reasons, first to ensure that no mistakes are made in producing the optimum result for the patient and also, since the treatment will take some time, to enable the dentist to fit a treatment into the appropriate appointments for the patient. Failure to plan usually leads to haphazard procedures such as restoring a tooth with an amalgam restoration then at a future appointment, when a partial denture is being constructed, realizing that a gold crown would have been a better restoration.

Diagnostic casts

The study of diagnostic casts is an essential part of the development of a treatment plan for patients requiring partial dentures and they must be an accurate reproduction of the teeth and adjacent tissues in a hard dental stone. The uses to which study casts can be put are listed in Table 8.1.

Table 8.1 Diagnostic casts

(1) Path of removal and insertion.
(2) Rest preparations.
(3) Embrasure clearance.
(4) Cuspal interference.
(5) Excessive contours requiring reduction.
(6) Acute angles that must be rounded.
(7) Retentive and non-retentive areas of abutment teeth.
(8) Creation of undercuts accomplished by discing or preparing dimples or grooves.
(9) Presentation of treatment plan to patient.
(10) Aid in determining order of progression of treatment.
(11) Fabrication of individual trays.
(12) Assist in preliminary design of partial denture.

However, one of the main uses is to examine the occlusion of the patient in detail. A correctly articulated cast will allow the occlusion to be examined from all positions, which is, of course, impossible when examining the patient. It is essential that the occlusion of the study models coincides with that of the patient and the centric occlusion should be no more than 1 mm anterior to the retruded contact position; movement from the retruded contact position should be in an anteroposterior direction without lateral deviation. Further, in lateral movements, the balancing cusps of the teeth should be completely out of contact when the working side teeth are in occlusion. For a more detailed discussion on occlusion the student is referred to the bibliography.

In those patients where centric occlusion and centric relation do not coincide correction of this anomaly must be undertaken as part of the treatment. This should, however, have been anticipated from the clinical examination and great care should have been taken in making the impressions, taking the jaw records and in mounting the casts if accurate results are to be achieved. Much academic argument exists depending on the definition of centric relation. In this instance, the most retruded position recorded (RP) is a terminal position sometimes referred to as the ligamentous position. This is a position which is usually 0–1 mm posterior to the centric occlusal position (muscular position). The muscular position normally coincides with centric occlusion.

The articulator is adjusted to give correct eccentric contacts and two methods are used.

(1) The opposing casts are positioned by means of wear facets on the teeth into right or left lateral eccentric positions and the articulator locked (see Figure 6.5).

(2) Interocclusal records are taken with the lower jaw protruded so that the incisor teeth are edge to edge and slightly apart. Interocclusal records may also be taken with the lower jaw in right and left lateral eccentric positions (Figure 8.1)

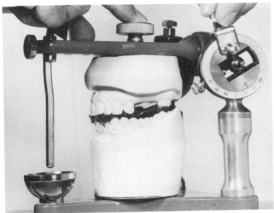

Figure 8.1 Eccentric records used to adjust the articular to give the correct lateral movement

The protrusive interocclusal record is placed between the casts and firmly held in place whilst the mechanism is locked. The results are checked by alternately placing the right and left lateral eccentric records between the casts and ensuring that the casts seat correctly. If the right lateral record is inserted, then the condylar mechanism on the left should be correct.

In some patients there is considerable bodily movement of the jaw during eccentric movement and this is called the 'Bennett movement' after Sir Norman Bennett (1958) who first recorded this particular shift of the mandible. This bodily movement of the mandible causes the condyle on the working side, which normally rotates, to move upwards, backwards and outwards, which on the articulator means that the condylar mechanism moves downwards, forwards and inwards. This movement is allowed for on the Dentatus and Hanau articulators by rotating the vertical pillars (see Figure 6.5) and also by withdrawing the screws in the anterior part of the condylar mechanism (Figure 6.5aK). The interocclusal records are now removed and the incisal guidance table (Figure 6.5) is adjusted to a position which will allow the upper incisor and canine teeth on the cast to move over the lower incisor teeth when the upper arm of the articulator is moved.

In many cases, however, where there is a deep overbite, this may not be possible and movement of the anterior segments over each other results in the posterior teeth separating.

The first and initial treatment is always to eliminate pain by temporary dressings or extraction of teeth and the stabilization of a patient's oral condition. In most cases also the teeth should be cleaned and polished as usually it is only after this procedure that an examination of the teeth for decay can be satisfactorily carried out.

Following this a decision must be made regarding the total care of the patient. If the teeth are very poor with gross decay and the alveolar ridges of reasonable shape, extraction of the remaining teeth and the construction of complete dentures may be indicated whilst in a very old person not in good health with a few sound teeth inactivity may be the best form of treatment. With the remaining patients, the younger patients will have all their remaining teeth whilst in later life many patients will have missing teeth and may possibly require a partial denture. This is not, however, an automatic procedure and restoration of missing teeth requires careful consideration.

For those who need a denture and are considered suitable the following sequence of events is suggested as a possible treatment plan.

(1) Any oral pathology must be eliminated. Inflamation often occurs beneath existing dentures. Treatment for this consists of use of drugs, such as nystatin or amphotericin B, which will eliminate the fungal condition in a few days or weeks.

(2) Any teeth which cannot be saved, unerupted teeth, and roots or cysts must be surgically treated. Roots that are covered with bone and asymptomatic with no evidence of associated pathology should be retained.

(3) If a partial denture is to be constructed then study casts as described in Chapter 3 are necessary and they must be surveyed in accordance with the principles outlined in Appendix IV.

Planning the type of partial denture required

Objectives

It is essential in planning the type of partial denture to be employed that the objectives of partial dentures be kept in mind and the denture which fulfils these objectives should be the simplest type possible. The objectives can best be demonstrated by studying the consequences of not providing a partial denture.

The consequences of failure to restore the loss of the natural teeth

In replacing the natural teeth with any form of partial denture in a way which will preserve the remaining teeth rather than destroy them, it is essential to understand the functions of such an appliance.

Drifting and tilting of the remaining natural teeth (Figure 8.2)

The lack of continuity of the dental arch allows the teeth to drift, tilt or rotate. The teeth are then not in ideal positions to receive the loads which are created in mastication and deterioration of the periodontal structures may take place. Also the tilting may lead to difficulty in keeping the teeth clean with consequent increased dental decay and periodontal disease.

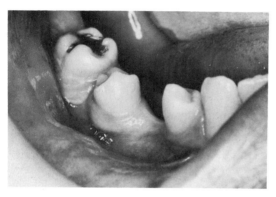

Figure 8.2 Drifting and rotation of the lower second premolar tooth

Overeruption (Figure 8.3)

When a natural tooth is unopposed it may overerupt. This may occur with or without alveolar bone growth and in the latter instance the periodontal structures deteriorate as the tooth is extruded while in the former case the excessive amount of

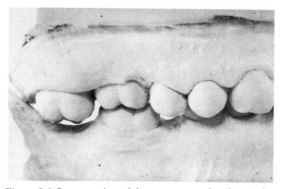

Figure 8.3 Overeruption of the upper second molar tooth due to lack of occlusal contact

alveolus may lead to difficulties if at a future time the patient requires complete dentures.

Reduction in masticatory efficiency

While reduced masticatory efficiency must occur as the natural teeth are lost or become functionless, this does not appear to be of importance to most patients today. Farrell (1956) has shown that a patient can digest an adequate diet with very little chewing.

Temporomandibular joint

Atypical chewing habits, overclosure, or an eccentric jaw relationship may occur following the loss of some natural teeth. This may lead to pain in the joint or its associated musculature (Figure 8.4).

Overloading of the supporting tissues

If the forces of mastication and occlusion are borne by a few remaining teeth this may lead to overloading, and consequent breakdown of the periodontal tissues with subsequent loss of the teeth. Failure to replace the posterior teeth by a partial

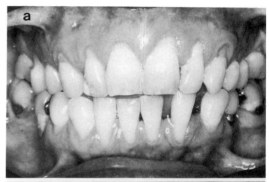

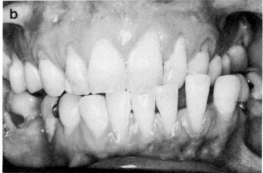

Figure 8.4 Eccentric jaw position in central occlusal leading to temporomandibular joint pain. (a) Jaw in centric relation, (b) in centric occlusion

denture, when the only remaining teeth are the six lower anteriors, leads to destruction of the alveolar bone of the premaxilla under an upper complete denture.

Defects of speech

Missing teeth often lead to speech defects. The most obvious are caused by the loss of an upper anterior tooth when 'lisping' results.

Loss of appearance

Missing upper anterior teeth reduce the overall pleasant appearance of the face, in the eyes of modern man. One of the most important reasons given by patients for wearing a denture is to improve their appearance.

Impaired oral hygiene

In addition to those factors mentioned in connection with the drifting and the tilting of the teeth, the loss of an opposing tooth prevents the natural abrasion of the surface of the remaining tooth which soon becomes covered with food debris. Under such conditions the risk of caries is increased.

Attrition (see Figure 1.1)

In some instances the periodontal membranes of teeth which are subjected to increased loads are not destroyed but remain healthy. The excessive loading then results in wear of the teeth with a reduced vertical dimension of the face when the teeth are in centric occlusion.

Effects on the soft tissues of the mouth

When teeth are lost the space in the dental arch becomes occupied by the soft tissues of the cheeks and tongue and if this continues for some years the patient may find it difficult to adapt to the wearing of an appliance which displaces these tissues.

Types of partial denture

A wide variety of different types of partial denture exist and are appropriate in different circumstances. For instance, if a large number of teeth are missing in the upper jaw with bounded saddles or the oral hygiene of the patient is far from satisfactory the Every denture (Figure 8.5) is an ideal form of restoration which can be made in either acrylic resin or metal. It is a very suitable denture for aesthetic restorations in young patients particularly where the teeth are not exposed to any great extent and with minimum guiding planes. It is, therefore, a very

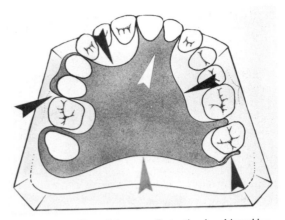

Figure 8.5 The 'Every' denture. Retention is achieved by restoration of contact points and as large a denture base as possible which does not encroach on the gingivae. Stability is obtained from the flanges and the saddle areas being as narrow as possible

'clean' design which will not prejudice the remaining teeth or gingival health.

The majority of partial dentures will be constructed in cobalt–chromium alloy though rarely cast gold may be indicated. The denture can be used to splint teeth and its retention can be achieved in a variety of ways. Even so the construction of a cast metal denture is expensive and would therefore only be contemplated for patients who have a reasonable satisfactory oral hygiene, although it has been shown that provided a patient is supervised with oral hygiene procedures and repeated encouragement and frequent recall appointments a partial denture can be successfully used for many years without detriment to the remaining oral tissues. The biggest problem lies in obtaining adequate retention and a number of alternative methods are employed as follows.

Clasps

The most common form of retention is that by using extracoronal clasps as part of the denture base casting. These types are discussed in detail in dealing with the design of a denture.

Swinglock partial denture

The swinglock partial denture (Figure 8.6) is extremely useful in situations where few teeth remain and undercuts are difficult to locate on the natural teeth and where it would be impossible to employ conventional clasping techniques. This type of denture is principally employed where a few remaining teeth exist. It suffers from the serious disadvantage of not being a particularly 'clean' type of design and is liable to collect considerable amounts of plaque on the denture and on the teeth.

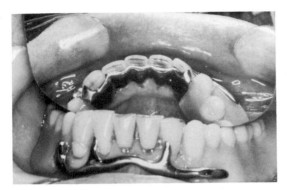

Figure 8.6 A swinglock partial denture

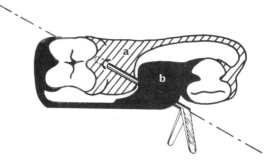

Figure 8.8 A sectional denture. Part a fits into the mesial undercut on the distal abutment and Part b into the distal undercut of the mesial abutment. The bolt is shown joining the two parts together

It has many advantages for those patients where spacing in the upper arch exists, or where a large amount of the root of the tooth is exposed when the labial bar can be covered in suitably stained acrylic resin to simulate the gum, creating a very pleasing result (Figure 8.7).

enough to withdraw the bolt from the posterior parts of the mouth.

Figure 8.8 demonstrates how the denture is constructed in two parts and a bolt used to join them together whilst Figure 8.9 shows a method for anterior teeth utilizing a split pin to hold the labial flange and the teeth in place which utilizes the undercuts on interproximal and labial surfaces of the teeth.

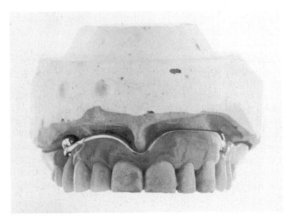

Figure 8.7 A swinglock partial using an acrylic flange

The hinge and the lock are commercially available in metal or plastic and these are incorporated into the wax pattern at the appropriate time and cast with the labial bar.

Sectional partial dentures

Sectional partial dentures are a very useful method of retaining a denture provided the surfaces of the teeth adjacent to the saddle have large undercuts which can be used to 'lock' the denture in place.

Two techniques are used which are reasonably easy from the constructional point of view, but using the bolt can be a problem for some patients with arthritic conditions since they are not dextrous

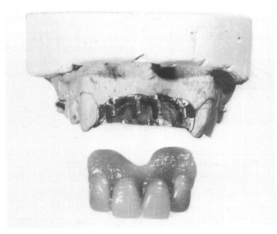

Figure 8.9 A sectional partial denture with a removable labial flange held in place by split pins

To achieve success with both types the two sections are made parallel to and inserted along guiding planes at divergent angles. The split pins are parallel to the labial surfaces of the anterior teeth whilst the metal based part is parallel and controlled by the guiding planes on the distal surfaces of posterior teeth. To achieve success these must be as divergent as possible. The advantages of the anterior flange in this denture are to give better aesthetics and good gingival contour which cannot be achieved by a conventional denture since the undercut areas involved are blocked out during construction, and when the denture is inserted a space is apparent at the gingival margin. The disadvantages of covering the gingival tissues with this type of denture is that if the oral hygiene is anything but excellent plaque accumulates on the teeth which leads to gingivitis and possible caries. This type of denture is an excellent one capable of a variety of designs and reference should be made to the text by L'Estrange and Pullen-Warner (1969).

Rotational path of insertion

Kroll (1981) has suggested that a compromise between the sectional denture and the normal clasp denture can be used. One end of the denture utilizes the undercut on the tooth adjacent to the saddle (Figure 8.10) and the remaining part of the denture rotates into place by conventional means. The advantages and disadvantages of this technique are shown in Table 8.2.

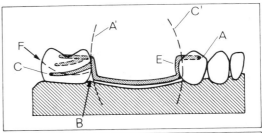

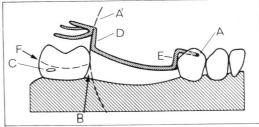

Figure 8.10 Diagram utilizing the undercut on one tooth and a rotational path of insertion. A' is the arc from centre A for seating the clasp and the minor connector D. B indicates the blocking out necessary. C' indicates the arc which the minor connector E must follow to be displaced as it rotates about point C. F is the survey line. (From Krol, 1981)

Table 8.2

Advantages of the rotational path
(1) Minimizes number of clasps.
(2) Anterior clasps may often be eliminated improving aesthetics.
(3) No distortion of rigid retentive component.
(4) May often be used in absence of lingual or buccal undercuts.
(5) Minimal tooth coverage.
(6) May be used in preference to an anterior fixed prosthesis to obtain better aesthetics.
(7) Easier to maintain oral hygiene.
(8) Minimal tooth preparation.

Disadvantages of rotational path
(1) No adjustment of rigid retentive component possible.
(2) Little tolerance for error.
(3) Requires well prepared occlusal or cingulum rests. May require conservative restorative treatment if dentine is exposed or to develop an acceptable rest seat.
(4) It is a removable prosthesis.

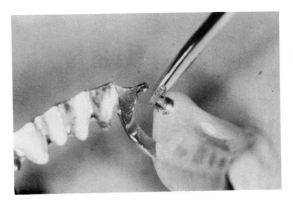

Figure 8.11 A partial denture providing a Z–A anchor

Z–A anchors

These are small spring-loaded plungers that can be utilized to engage small depressions in restorations and can be very effective when used in the anterior part of the mouth to create retention without the unaesthetic appearance of clasps on the canine tooth (Figure 8.11). If natural undercuts exist on the teeth the enamel surface can be slightly modified and the retainer used without a restoration but this is not as satisfactory as if a depression can be created in a restoration. This type of anchor does not require any difference in the constructional method of the metal denture since it is inserted into the acrylic resin of the saddle.

Precision attachments

Precision attachments are usually two precision components which are manufactured to form an articulated joint. They are designed to replace the occlusal rest, bracing arm, and retaining arm of a conventional clasped partial denture. They are generally smaller and machined to fine tolerances and much more efficient in resisting the forces applied to a denture than are the conventional parts of a clasping unit.

They have the advantage that:

(1) They give better retention and stability than clasps.
(2) There is less food stagnation.
(3) They are less liable to fracture than clasps.
(4) They are more aesthetic than clasps.
(5) They are less bulky and more pleasant for the patient.
(6) Multiple abutments are often necessary and if the teeth are slightly mobile due to previous periodontal disease they will be splinted together by the crowns on the teeth. This is thus a rigid splint and more successful than a removable one.

In order to produce a satisfactory result, however, preparation of the abutment teeth must be made to produce adequate retainers. The teeth must be large enough to accommodate the selected attachments and the clinical time taken and the laboratory work make the total restoration extremely expensive. The clasped partial denture or the two-part partial denture will, therefore, remain the main type of removable denture for the majority of patients because it requires the minimum of clinical and laboratory time. Precision attachments need not,

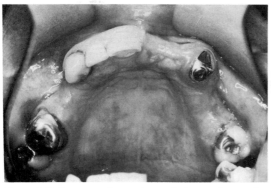

Figure 8.12 An eccentric attachment being used to retain a partial denture

however, be very 'precise' and the term 'precision' is not an ideal one. For instance, the eccentric attachment (Figure 8.12) does not need elaborate equipment and can be fitted with an ordinary surveyor. Several manufacturers make a range of attachments and, therefore, the total number of attachments available is exceedingly large. Many are, however, very similar and if the design of a partial denture is understood the selection of the attachment will not cause concern. In fact, most practitioners only use a small number of attachments.

Preliminary design of the partial denture

Once the type of denture has been decided upon the actual stages in drawing up the design are carried out. The procedure for this is dealt with in Chapter 10.

(1) Once the design has been established the decision on the type of restorations and mouth preparation can be planned as outlined in Chapter 11. Restorations not involved with the partial denture can also be planned on the merits of the tooth itself and the amount of tissue to be destroyed together with its position within the oral cavity. Anterior restorations are usually made with composite materials because of their natural tooth colour whilst posterior teeth may be restored with amalgam or gold.
(2) Peridontal treatment must also be planned. This can be carried out at any stage and may involve surgical removal of tissue, deep scaling or drug therapy to eliminate infection. In some instances when an existing partial denture is involved it may be necessary to leave this treatment until a new partial denture has been constructed.
(3) In rare instances, orthodontics may be required to move teeth into a more favourable position to create better aesthetics or upright the teeth to give better support for a partial denture or a bridge.
(4) The last procedure is to construct the partial denture.

Having established a complete plan of the patient's treatment it can be activated in a logical sequence.

9

The function of the component parts of a partial denture

Before beginning the design of a partial denture it is essential to understand the forces which can be applied to the denture during the acts of chewing, swallowing and speech. The magnitude of the forces will naturally vary considerably according to the age and sex of the patient, since these factors affect the development of the muscles of mastication. An understanding of the means used to resist these forces and to support the partial denture is the basis of partial denture design.

Occlusal/vertical forces

These forces should be distributed to the natural teeth as widely as possible since, under these conditions, the load is distributed by the periodontal membrane to a large area of bone. The transmission of these forces from the denture to the tooth is achieved through an occlusal, incisal or cingulum rest (Figures 9.1 and 11.5).

Where a natural tooth is present at each end of an edentulous space and the root area of the teeth is sufficient to support the extra load an entirely tooth-supported denture is possible. As a general rule, the root area of the abutment teeth should be the same as that of the teeth which have been lost. In this situation, if the periodontal condition of the teeth, and all other factors, are satisfactory a fixed bridge could be constructed. But if conditions are not suitable for a bridge then a partial denture may be constructed provided its design is carefully considered.

Where abutment teeth are not adequate to support an entirely tooth-supported denture, or where there is only one supporting tooth, the denture must either be supported by the mucous membrane and the underlying bone, or by a combination of the teeth and the mucous membrane. A combined support, as in a free-end saddle, may lead to damage to the periodontal membrane of the abutment tooth due to the compressibility of the mucous membrane allowing the denture to move laterally or anteroposteriorly during function (Figure 9.2). This rocking of the tooth can be prevented if the design and construction of the partial denture is carried out with great care.

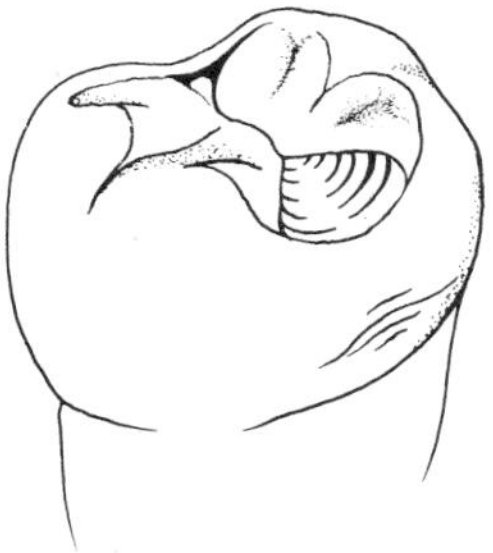

Figure 9.1 Illustration of occlusal rest seat

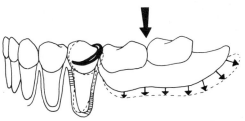

Figure 9.2 The effect of an occlusal load on a free-end saddle is to cause sinking of the saddle, rotation of the tooth with changes in pressure in the periodontal membrane

Only in the upper jaw, where a large area of palatal bone is available, can a denture be entirely supported by the mucous membrane. A denture of this type is shown in Figure 8.5. Resorption of palatal bone does not occur since the load is widely distributed on the palatal processes of the maxillae which are normally subjected to pressure from the tongue. The load from the denture, therefore, increases the normal force upon the bone, but since it is of the same type, i.e. compressive, the bone can withstand this extra load as long as it is within physiological limits.

Saddles

These are the parts of the denture which replace the lost alveolar bone and the teeth. When the patient chews food on the artificial teeth, the forces must be transmitted to the oral tissues. If the saddle is tooth-supported at each end (bounded saddles) the area of the saddle is unimportant and can be as small as is practicable. In the case of saddles without a posterior tooth (free-end saddles) support must come from the soft tissues and the alveolar bone, together with the tooth at the anterior end of the saddle. It is, therefore, essential to reduce the forces on the alveolar bone as much as possible to prevent its resorption, and therefore the free-end saddle should be as large as possible, covering all non-movable tissue.

Horizontal lateral forces

Lateral forces are applied to the teeth and the mucous membranes when the lower jaw moves from

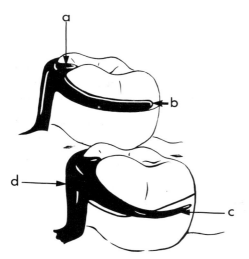

Figure 9.3 Clasping unit showing the component parts (a) occlusal rest, (b) bracing arm, (c) retentive arm, and (d) minor connector

side to side with teeth in contact, thus causing the denture to move. These lateral movements of the partial denture are transmitted to the teeth and the supporting structures by those parts of the denture fitting on either side of the teeth (Figure 9.3) and called bracing arms. These parts of the denture are placed on or above the survey lines (see Appendix IV), generally on the lingual or palatal surfaces of the teeth. That part of the retaining arm or clasp which is above the survey line is also rigid, and will provide considerable resistance to lateral forces.

Lateral forces will cause movement of the teeth and compression of the periodontal membrane which may lead to resorption of bone, particularly since the forces may be large and the area of supporting bone small. It is thus advisable to reduce the pressure on the hard tissues to a minimum by distributing these horizontal forces to as many teeth as possible.

Since the bracing arm is on or above the survey line, it will disengage from the tooth when the denture is withdrawn, whilst the clasping arm will still be exerting force on the tooth (Figure 9.4)

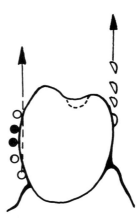

Figure 9.4 When reciprocation is not at the level of the retaining arm a lateral force is exerted on the tooth

during the removal of the denture. Ideally, the clasp arm, when flexed in this way, should have a supporting arm for the other side of the tooth to prevent the periodontal ligament from being damaged. In order that the function of bracing and reciprocation are effective, it would be necessary for the bracing arm to be at the same level as the tip of the clasp arm. This is seldom possible unless the tooth is severely ground or a restoration, such as a gold crown, is made with a specially prepared guiding plane on the lingual side parallel to the path of insertion (Figure 9.5).

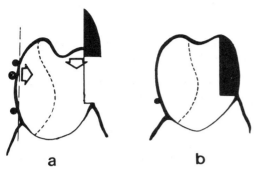

Figure 9.5 A bracing arm recessed into a gold crown giving reciprocation in all positions of the retaining arm. a, on insertion; b, fully seated

Horizontal anteroposterior forces

Forward and backward movements of the lower jaw with the teeth in contact will result in possible movement of the denture if not resisted by standing teeth or by the bracing arms and clasps which pass around the teeth.

In a bounded saddle, they will be resisted by the teeth themselves. In the case of an anterior saddle, additional resistance is also obtained by clasps passing round the teeth. The free-end saddle is prevented from moving under these forces by clasps and also by the shape of the ridges. Clasping arms, to be effective, must be more than half way around the abutment tooth.

In the lower, the retromolar pad, and in the upper, the tuberosity will also give some resistance to those forces moving the denture.

Vertical displacing forces

During mastication, sticky foods will adhere to the artificial teeth attached to the saddle of the denture and when the jaws are opened the denture will be moved away from the seated position. To prevent this, flexible arms are added to the denture which engage areas of the teeth that are undercut relative to the displacement path (see Appendix IV). The force required to bend the flexible arms sufficiently to pass over the most bulbous part of the tooth should be greater than the force produced by the sticky foods when the jaw is opened.

The resisting force of the clasp will depend upon its features:

(1) The depth of the undercut engaged.
(2) The cross-sectional shape and size of the clasp.
(3) The modulus of elasticity of the alloy.
(4) The length of the clasp arm.

(5) The position of the clasp arm in relation to the force applied.
(6) The angle of the incline plane of the tooth surface.
(7) The frictional resistance between the enamel and the clasp arm.
(8) The mobility of the tooth.

Rotational displacement

So far, only the vertical displacing forces have been considered, but in the case of the free-end saddle any force displacing the saddle will tend to cause rotation about tips of the direct retaining arms (i.e. clasps) and these points, when joined by an imaginary line, form a rotational axis. In order to stabilize the denture against rotational forces, an occlusal rest placed on the opposite side of the axis to the force causing the displacement will, whilst the direct retainers are effective, tend to hold the saddle in place (Figure 9.6). The effectiveness of the system

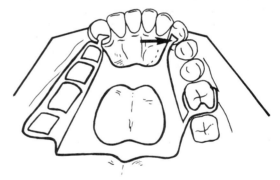

Figure 9.6 An indirect retainer

depends on the distance between the indirect retainer as it is called, and the fulcrum axis and the distance between the applied force and the fulcrum axis. For maximum effectiveness, these distances should be equal (Figure 9.7). However, where the distance from the axis to the indirect retainer is small and the distance from the applied force to the axis is large, the mechanical effectiveness of such a device will be minimal and its addition to the denture must therefore be questioned. This is discussed in more detail in the next chapter.

Connectors

Once all the forces have been considered, it is necessary to join the parts of the denture together since this helps distribute the stresses, particularly

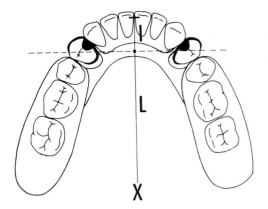

Figure 9.7 A fulcrum axis is most effective when (I) and (L) are equal. As (I) gets smaller in relation to (L) the less effective will be the indirect retention

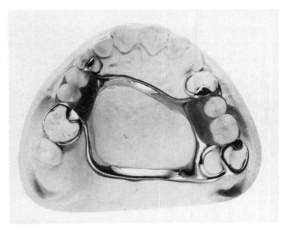

Figure 9.8 Palatal connector joining the parts of the denture together

horizontal ones, which cause more damage to the periodontal membrane of the teeth than vertical forces. By joining the pieces together with bars or plates (Figure 9.8) the forces applied to one side of the denture in the mouth are automatically transmitted to the other side, thus reducing the forces of the

teeth on the chewing side considerably. Further, when all are connected together the denture is quite large and it is then impossible to inhale it or swallow it. This is an important factor since there have been a number of reported deaths as a result of inhalation of small dentures.

10

Design of partial dentures

A systematic approach

The stages in developing the design of a partial denture should be approached systematically and each stage produced in response to the conditions that exist for the patient. Preconceived designs which may be used for all patients exhibiting the same general features are doomed to failure. As each stage is completed, it should be drawn on a design sheet or work card and on the diagnostic casts to help the laboratory technician.

Stage 1: classification of the support for each saddle

A decision must be made on how each saddle is to be classified with regard to its support when the saddle is subject to occlusal forces. It can be either entirely supported by the natural teeth, i.e. a bounded saddle, or entirely supported by the soft tissues and underlying bone. In many instances, as in free-end saddles, some support is derived from both of these.

Tooth-supported and bounded saddles (Beckett Classes I and III)

Several factors must be taken into account when planning the support for the saddle of the denture. The principal ones are:

(1) The periodontal condition of the remaining teeth.
(2) The number and situation of the missing teeth.
(3) The nature of the opposing teeth, i.e. artificial or natural.
(4) The nature of any supporting soft tissues.

(5) The length of the edentulous space.
(6) The masticatory effort which the individual naturally uses in comminuting the food.
(7) Aesthetics.

Bounded saddles have advantages over free-end saddles in that the number of displacing paths are reduced and therefore the retention of the denture will be improved and the saddles will not move about under occlusal loads to the same extent as free-end saddles. The tooth-supported saddle only becomes a problem when it is lengthened to such an extent that the periodontal support is too small for the occlusal load. This occurs, for instance, when the abutment teeth are a lateral incisor at one end and a second or third molar at the other end and in such circumstances one must consider alternative means of support.

Saddles supported by the mucous membrane (Class II)

When it is impossible to support a saddle on the teeth it must be supported by the mucous membrane and one way, already suggested, is to construct an entirely mucosal supported upper denture; if this is not possible one must attempt to 'divide' the load between the mucosa and the periodontum. This problem of 'dividing' the load is a difficult one and has led to a great deal of thought and many ingenious devices to achieve this aim. Ultimately, they all lead to loading the mucous membrane and attempting to stabilize the saddle from rocking around the abutment tooth. The principal means of attempting to provide a distribution of the load on the supporting tissue in this type of case are by one of the following techniques.

Reducing the occlusal load

This may be achieved by reducing the number or the occlusal surface area of the teeth on the denture.

Distribution of load between the teeth and the mucous membrane

This can be attempted by:

(1) Special impression techniques whereby a negative likeness of the tissues is achieved while they are under load.
(2) By the placing of occlusal rests away from the saddle in order to allow the saddle to sink more evenly into the tissues which therefore increases the load on the mucosa compared with the periodontium. It also reduces the torque on the supporting tooth. This technique also requires an impression to be taken with the mucosa under load (see Chapter 13).

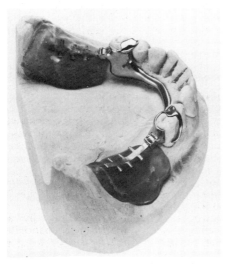

Figure 10.1 A hinge stress breaker on a free-end saddle denture

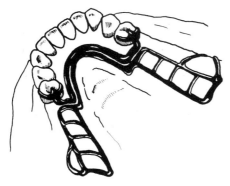

Figure 10.2 A bilateral free-end saddle denture with a split connector to allow stress breaking

(3) The use of stress-breaking devices, such as hinges or flexible connectors joining the saddles to the clasps (Figures 10.1 and 10.2). These types of design are complicated, are prone to breaking and there is evidence to demonstrate that they do not give as successful long-term results as rigid designs so are becoming less used than previously.

Distributing the load widely

This implies increasing the saddle to its largest possible area and using as much occlusal support as possible.

Once the decision regarding the support for the saddle against occlusal forces has been made, it is possible to outline the periphery of the saddles on the study casts and place occlusal rests in their correct positions to support the saddles.

Siting the occlusal rests

Occlusal rests have the following functions.

(1) To support the denture against the vertical forces of occlusion and transmit these forces to the natural teeth.
(2) If the rest is prepared as a box which fits into a specially prepared cavity in an inlay or in a tooth, it transmits horizontal forces to the teeth.
(3) To deflect food and prevent packing between the saddle and the tooth.
(4) They may be used as onlays to improve the occlusion.
(5) They may act as indirect retainers.

In general terms, a Class I saddle (bounded) is supported by rests adjacent to the saddle. The force transmitted to the tooth will depend upon the position of the load in relation to the occlusal rest. If, midway between the rests, equal load would be transmitted to each tooth and if one tooth is weaker than the other in terms of support, consideration should be given to moving the rest on the weaker tooth further from the point of application of the load. It has been shown that most chewing takes place in the first molar area and, assuming this premise, it is possible to adjust the position of the rest to gain the best support.

A further consideration concerns the position of the occlusal rest on the tooth. For instance, if the occlusal rest is on an inclined plane and at an angle to the long axis of the teeth, the occlusal forces will tend to cause movement of the tooth away from the rest, and it is for this reason that some adjustment of the tooth surface is necessary to ensure that forces are directed parallel to the long axis of the tooth. Consideration of the method of preparing teeth to allow for this situation will be discussed in Chapter 11. Under normal circumstances, however carefully this is considered, the siting of the rest can seldom

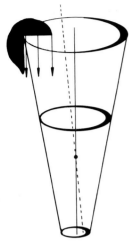

Figure 10.3 Tipping action of an occlusal rest on a tooth

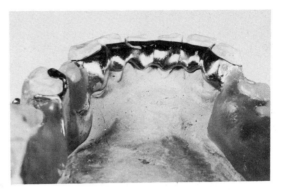

Figure 10.4 A connector used to give indirect retention and also bracing. This type of connector is a strengthened Kennedy continuous clasp and is commonly called a dental bar

(unless it is an onlay) direct the forces straight down the long axis of the tooth as the tooth itself is approximately conical in shape (Figure 10.3). In a bounded saddle the tooth is prevented from moving by the saddle and the opposing force from its counterpart at the opposing end of the saddle. In a free-end saddle, however, this movement may occur with nothing to stop the tooth tipping towards the edentulous area. For this reason, and for other considerations discussed in relation to clasps, the rest is always placed on the mesial side of the abutment tooth with free-end saddles, thus causing any tooth movement to be towards the adjacent natural tooth. In some instances of tipped teeth, or where a wide area of support is needed, two rests are employed on either end of the tooth, thus reciprocating the torque effect of one occlusal rest and transmitting the forces along the long axis of the tooth. This is particularly evident in lower molar teeth which are often tilted.

Stage II: the provision of bracing arms

The prevention of movement in a horizontal plane and the distribution of horizontal forces to the natural teeth, takes place via the bracing arms (sometimes called reciprocating arms). These are placed on all the abutment teeth on or above the survey lines, and are joined to the occlusal rests. In order to reduce the load on any one tooth it may be necessary to include more teeth than those adjacent to the saddles, particularly so if the number of teeth are small or weakened by previous periodontal disease.

Bracing also occurs in an anteroposterior and lateral direction from connectors which are placed on the teeth (Figure 10.4).

The rigid part of a retaining arm which is above the survey line may also provide some bracing and the clasping unit, as a whole, prevents movement in all directions.

Stage III: direct retention

Many types of retaining arms have been advocated and called after their originators but, provided the basic rules are followed, knowing the names of the clasps is not important.

(1) The clasp arms must always be associated with an occlusal rest so that they are maintained in a constant position.
(2) A retentive arm is always opposed by a reciprocating arm and together more than half the circumference of the tooth must be enclosed in the clasping unit.
(3) The clasp arms must be as small as possible and fitted in such a way that they will not trap food or lead to unnecessary plaque accumulation.

Clasps may be divided into two main types; those which approach the undercut from the gingival surface (Figure 10.5) and those which approach from an occlusal surface shown in Figure 9.3. For a more thorough analysis of clasp design the reader is referred to the works of Blatterfein (1951) and Demer (1976).

The retention obtained by the clasps is, however, variable and thus the design of the clasp must be considered with care.

Depth of undercut

The amount of force necessary to flex the cantilever arm can be varied by changing the position of the tip

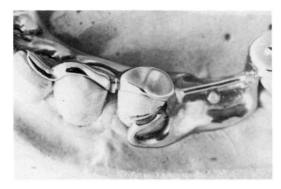

Figure 10.5 A Roach C type gingivally approaching clasp arm

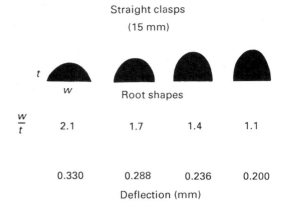

Figure 10.7 The effect of clasp cross-sectional shape on deflection of the clasp tip in cobalt–chromium alloy clasps

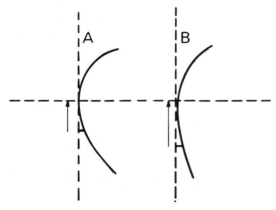

Figure 10.6 Retention can be varied by increasing the horizontal depth of the undercut used but is also dependent on the vertical movement necessary to cause disengagement of the clasp

of the clasp, as in Figure 10.6. The horizontal undercut depth is the important consideration, but the vertical displacement before reaching the survey line is also of some importance since it will necessitate the application of the displacing force for a longer period of time to displace the denture. During chewing this may not happen, and only short periods of high load will occur, and will be insufficient in terms of time to displace the denture if the displacing path is a long one.

The cross-sectional shape, size and length of the clasp arm

Clasps vary in cross-sectional shape, and also in actual dimensions, depending upon the type of preformed wax or plastic pattern employed in the construction. The flexibility will vary, depending

upon the shape, as shown in Figure 10.7, where the deflection recorded is at the proportional limit and when the clasp is straight.

Bending the clasp stiffens it considerably, particularly so if it passes around more than half the tooth surface. However, such a procedure automatically lengthens the arm and an increase in the deflection will take place which is usually in a cubic relationship. Doubling the length of a clasp, therefore, will cause an eight-fold increase in the deflection. When a fixed deflection is used, however, it may mean that with increased flexibility less retention is obtained as smaller forces will cause the same amount of displacement of the clasp and, generally, when considering long clasps, the depth of undercut can be increased.

The modulus of elasticity of the alloy

The modulus of elasticity of a cobalt–chromium alloy is twice that of gold alloy. For a given load, therefore, the clasp in the base metal alloy will flex only half that of the noble metal, given that the dimensions of the clasps are the same. In constructing clasps, therefore, the undercut used for cobalt–chromium alloys should be half that of gold. Generally, the amount used is 0.25 mm for the cobalt–chromium alloys. Less than this is not practicable owing to the inaccuracies of the casting process and more exerts too great a force on the tooth which may lead to damage to the periodontal membrane. An alternative technique is to use a clasp of smaller cross-section for the cobalt–chromium alloys than for gold, but this has some disadvantages in that it is weaker and more likely to be broken or deformed by the patient, and also small flaws or porosities in the casting are more likely to occur and will lead to fracture.

The best approach to this problem is to design, where possible, long cobalt–chromium clasps and use a slightly greater undercut, 0.35 mm if possible. In those situations where it is imperative to use a short arm with a cobalt–chromium base, a gold wire clasp should be used and soldered to the base. If a gold casting is being made, the casting itself may be used to form the clasp, but if there is doubt, a wire clasp would again be preferable as the wrought structure has better mechanical properties. Fabricated wire clasps have, however, some disadvantages in the lack of accuracy of fit to the tooth.

The angles of approach of the clasp arm

It has been said that the angle at which a clasp arm slides over the tooth during its displacement affects the amount of retention obtained. This so-called trip action has been likened to a fountain pen being pushed or pulled over a writing pad. As the angle of the pen approaches a right angle we receive a sensation of tripping action when the pen is pushed forward over the pad, but this is entirely absent when the pen is pulled across the pad. This effect has never been satisfactorily explained in relation to the clasp arm.

To some extent the situation will also vary with the convexity of the tooth surface. In very bulbous teeth the undercut used will be close to the survey line and the vertical movement of the clasp small on the displacement. The inclined plane of the tooth surface will, therefore, be greater with respect to the clasp and thus it is said the retention will be increased.

The position of the clasp in relation to the displacing force

The position of the clasp tip and the fulcrum axis to the applied load is of importance in retention. The system is similar to a class 1 lever, and the nearer the clasp tip is to the load, the better will be the retention. This is particularly important in the case of a free-end saddle and retention in the case of conventional clasping (Figure 9.2) will be less than that when the rest is placed on the mesial part of the tooth and the clasp tips are placed as near the saddles as possible (Figure 10.8). A similar argument can be put forward in relation to bounded saddles and, where possible, tips of clasps should always be placed as near the saddle as possible and, generally speaking, it will be found that owing to resorption of the alveolar ridge, the undercuts on the teeth are usually found adjacent to the saddles.

Aesthetics is one situation which prevents this approach being used since the patients do not like to show clasps on their anterior teeth. A typical example of this is seen in Figure 10.21 as the clasps have been moved to posterior teeth thus rendering them less effective.

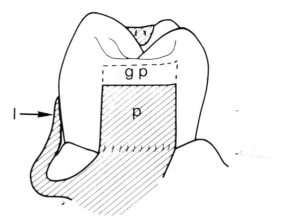

Figure 10.8 The preferable arrangement of the clasp tip as near the saddle as possible and used in conjunction with a mesial rest and a distal plate (p). This is commonly called the RPI system, i.e. rest, plate and I bar. gp is guiding plane produced by grinding the tooth surface (From Krol, 1981)

Mobility of teeth

It has already been explained in relation to Figure 9.4 that unless the bracing arm is also a reciprocating arm, pressure will be applied to the tooth when the denture is withdrawn. If the tooth is slightly mobile and is capable of movement in the same order as the depth of the undercut used, the tooth may well move rather than the clasp bend. The tooth will move under loads far less than those required to cause flexure of the clasp arm, and if there is doubt about the tooth then either a true reciprocating arm should be used, or a very flexible wire retaining arm.

In the early days of partial denture construction, wire clasps were used which had a spring action in gripping the tooth. It was for this reason that reciprocating arms were employed since it was possible to obtain orthodontic tooth movement with this type of clasp. With present-day techniques, where the casting is in a passive state when the denture is seated, the use of reciprocating arms appears to be less essential but, ideally, both reciprocating and bracing should be combined in one arm.

The relative merits of occlusally and gingivally approaching clasps

Bracing and retention

It is claimed that gingivally approaching clasps produce more friction with the enamel and are more retentive than occlusally approaching ones. However, in general, the gingival clasp arm is longer and often more flexible and, on the whole, less retentive than the occlusally approaching clasp. Consequently, the gingivally approaching clasp is less useful for bracing since the whole of the arm is flexible.

Damage to the oral tissues

The gingivally approaching clasp has been shown to be potentially more likely to create gingival pathology. Further, the area of food stagnation is at the neck of the tooth and the cementum in this area is more likely to be affected by caries than enamel. Trauma to the gingivae is also likely to occur with gingivally approaching clasps, unless carefully relieved. Patients often remove their dentures by putting their fingernails below the clasps and exerting considerable force; deformation and damage to the soft tissues may occur by mishandling in this way.

Aesthetics

Whilst it is not possible to make hard and fast rules concerning clasps, it is generally found that the gingivally approaching clasp is to be preferred for aesthetic reasons. However, where a large amount of gingivae is shown on smiling, the gingivally approaching clasp may be more noticeable than the occlusally approaching variety.

Retention can also be obtained by other methods which have been described in Chapter 8 but the principles of stress distribution still apply and occlusal rests, bracing arms, etc. are still necessary.

Stage IV: indirect retention

The basic concepts of indirect retention have already been discussed. This will become more evident when the principles of design are applied to a specific situation. Indirect retention is obviously of greater moment in the upper jaw since gravity is applied to the denture at all times, and there is, therefore, a constant displacing force on saddles which is not applicable to the lower denture. It is for this reason that, in many instances, indirect retainers are omitted from lower dentures.

The various types of indirect retainers used depend primarily upon the tolerance of the patient to additional extensions from the denture and, where possible, it is preferable to minimize the use of these additional parts of the denture. It is always a wise policy to make the denture as simple as possible.

When used in the upper jaw it is sometimes difficult, on the anterior teeth, to ensure sufficient room for the thickness of the metal, and also, in the anterior part of the mouth, the extension of the denture may cause difficulties with speech.

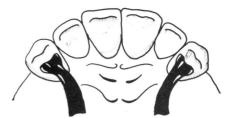

Figure 10.9 Cummer indirect retainers

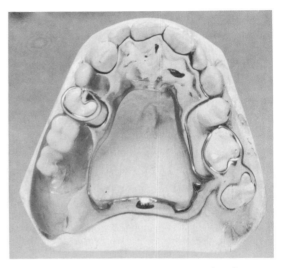

Figure 10.10 The palatal plate connector acting also as an indirect retainer

The simplest form of indirect retainer is the occlusal rest, sometimes referred to as the Cummer rest (Figure 10.9). However, in order to avoid the problems of tolerance with this type of extension, it is often converted into a plate covering the backs of the teeth (Figure 10.10) and thus forms the major connector. In some cases, the bars of the denture also help stability, although the soft tissues are poor in this respect. The anterior palatal bar may be used for upper free-end saddles and the posterior palatal bars for anterior restorations.

Stage V: connectors
Major connectors

The major connectors are of the following types.

Maxilla

(1) Anterior and posterior palatal bar/strap.
(2) Single palatal bar/strap.
(3) Palatal horseshoe.
(4) Palatal plate.

Mandible

(1) Lingual bar and sublingual bar.
(2) Buccal bar.
(3) Lingual plate.
(4) Dental bar.

Maxillary connectors

A major connector is that part of a partial denture which joins all the parts of the prosthesis together. It is essential to have the connectors 'rigid' in order to transmit the forces developed during function to all supporting structures of the mouth. Since the forces which occur during function are difficult to measure, it is not possible to define the dimensions of connectors precisely in order to ensure that they are 'rigid' and not flexible. Certain sizes of bar or plate are, however, in common use and in the absence of more detailed knowledge it is wise to follow these since they have been shown to be successful.

A major connector should be located away from the moving tissues and at the same time avoid impinging on gingival tissues. Ideally, the connectors should be at least 3 mm from the gingival margins and on insertion of the denture the connectors must not irritate the soft tissues when moving over them. This particularly applies to a lingual or buccal bar which, on insertion, passes over the gingival margins to reach its final position. Where connectors come in contact with the natural teeth, it is essential to support the connector to prevent movement and gingival irritation and it must be shaped so as to be continuous with the tissues and avoid irritation to the tongue. This is of particular importance in the anterior palatal region, where irregularities irritate the tip of the tongue. Plates should be made as thin as possible, but without weakening the denture unduly, and the edges should be blended into the tissues.

Minor connectors

These are small struts which join rests and clasps to the major connector. They should be as unobtrusive as possible and fit between the teeth and cross the minimum of gingival surface. Strength is important since they support the denture against the occlusal forces and therefore transmit heavy loads to the natural teeth.

It will be seen, therefore, that in the completed design the various parts of the denture help to resist the various forces which attempt to cause movement of the appliance and that, where possible, these forces are distributed over as wide an area of the natural tissues as possible.

The single midpalatal bar/strap

It is not always easy to differentiate between what are called bars and plates, but since the objective is to have a rigid structure and, at the same time, make it tolerable for the patient, the term 'bar' includes those connectors which are rather wider than one might anticipate (Figure 10.11). This type of connector is probably the most readily tolerated of palatal connectors, being in the middle of the palate and causing less interference with the tongue than any other type. This connector also usually lies within the confines of the occlusal rests and, therefore, rocking of the denture is less likely when pressed upon by the tongue.

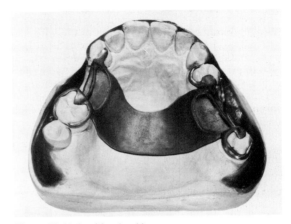

Figure 10.11 A mid-palatal bar

Anterior palatal bar

This bar lies on the rugae, and is in an area where the tip of the tongue touches the palate during speech. Phonetic difficulties and lack of tolerance are problems with this type of bar which should be avoided whenever possible. It is only used when long saddles are not sufficiently rigid with a posterior or mid-palatal bar and the denture is then converted into a 'ring' design (Figure 10.12).

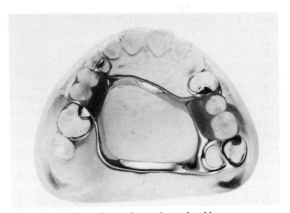

Figure 10.12 Posterior and anterior palatal bars

Present-day designs would tend to convert this into a plate design rather than use two bars, since modern impression and casting techniques enable a casting to be made with a high degree of accuracy. The cost of the cobalt–chromium alloy is not an important part of the total cost of the denture, and the design, therefore, need not be related to the amount of alloy used. When gold castings are being considered then, obviously, the design would require the use of a minimum amount of alloy.

Posterior palatal bar/strap (Figure 10.13)

This is similar in size to the mid-palatal bar and is normally positioned at the junction of the hard and soft palate, just anterior to the vibrating line. It is most commonly used when free-end saddles exist; it is well tolerated by the tongue and is said to act as an indirect retainer, but owing to the compressibility of the tissues, this action can only be minimal. A careful impression technique is required and a high degree of technical skill, since sometimes it is found that the bar does not fit accurately on to the palate. In most cases the cause can be attributable to metal shrinkage or to an inadequate impression.

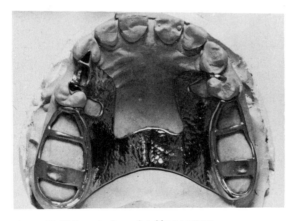

Figure 10.13 A posterior palatal bar or strap

Palatal horsehoe type connectors

This type of design is satisfactory if anterior saddles are involved, but it should never be used as in Figure 10.14. Here the force on the saddles tends to separate the posterior parts of the denture and, therefore, exerts torque on abutment teeth and a midline stress in the connector. This presents problems since the plate must be thin to prevent irritation of the tongue, and the whole structure is, therefore, not rigid enough. In this case, a midpalatal bar or strap should be used, or a 'ring' design with posterior and anterior palatal bars.

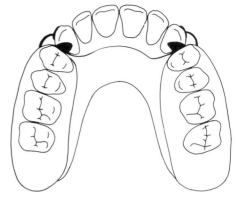

Figure 10.14 A palatal 'horseshoe' connector

Palatal plates

The disadvantage of these is the additional tissue covered, but they are advantageous in that they can be made of any material, give extra support to the denture and, if retention is a problem, this is augmented by the pressure from the tongue on the palatal connector, which helps to hold the denture in place. An example of this type of connector is seen in Figure 10.15.

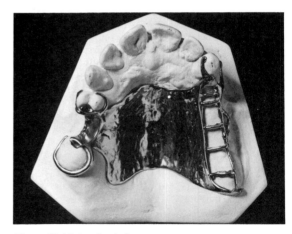

Figure 10.15 A palatal plate connector

Mandibular connectors

The lingual bar

Lingual bars are usually placed on the wall of the alveolus 2–3 mm below the gingival margins (see Figure 10.16). They must not impinge on moving soft tissue and should be supported so that movement will not cause compression of the mucosal tissues. Usually a relief is provided so that rotation of bar on loading will not cause tissue trauma.

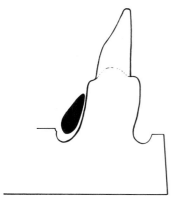

Figure 10.16 The position of a lingual bar in relation to the alveolus and the floor of the mouth

Patients often find it difficult to tolerate lingual bars and casts, rather than wrought bars, well adapted to the tissues, are essential. Problems arise in those patients where there is inadequate space between the floor of the mouth and the gingivae. These problems may be dealt with in a number of ways, as follows.

The sublingual bar The sublingual bar is much better tolerated than an ordinary lingual bar since it lies very low in the floor of the mouth (Figure 10.17). It does, however, require considerable expertise in obtaining the correct impression. It is shorter than an ordinary lingual bar and its thickness is greatest in the horizontal plane and, therefore, it is much more rigid than an ordinary lingual bar.

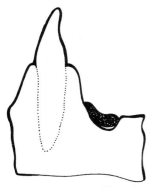

Figure 10.17 The position of a sublingual bar

The lingual plate A further method of overcoming the shortage of space between the floor of the mouth and the gingivae is to use a complete lingual plate (see Figure 12.15). These are thin metal castings with no discontinuities which join the saddles together and are, therefore, extremely well tolerated. They combine indirect retention as well as being connectors, but they have the disadvantage of covering the gingival tissues and the interdental spaces. These are, therefore, not to be recommended unless the oral hygiene of the patient is very good. They can also provide certain difficulties for those patients who do not return for repeated rebasing of the dentures as the lower part of the lingual plate will move forward and may cause tissue irritation.

A modified 'continuous clasp' – dental bar In recent years the thickened continuous clasp has been developed which is well tolerated by the patients and does not require careful impression procedures, such as the sublingual bar. It overcomes the problem of covering the gingival tissues and, if properly constructed, is of adequate rigidity as a connector. This is probably the most useful connector for the lower jaw since it has few disadvantages apart from covering the natural teeth (see Figure 10.4).

A buccal or labial bar These bars are similar to lingual bars, but are used when the teeth are so lingually inclined that all other connectors are impossible to design. Being longer than lingual bars, they must, naturally, be thicker to obtain the necessary rigidity and, ideally, should be cast in cobalt–chromium alloy to give the greatest stiffness for the minimum amount of bulk. They lie in exactly the same relationship to the gingivae as the lingual bar, i.e. 2–3 mm below the gingival margins and extend down into the buccal sulcus. They are so seldom used that it is impossible to comment on whether they are well tolerated by patients (Figure 10.18).

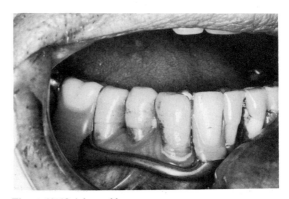

Figure 10.18 A buccal bar

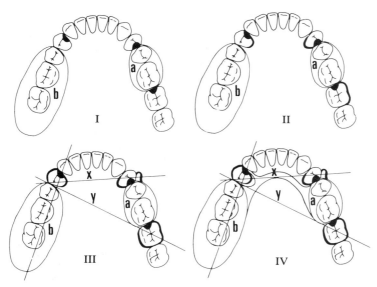

Figure 10.19 Case 1. Stages in the design of a lower denture with a bounded or free-end saddle (Kennedy Class II modification I)

A systematic approach to partial denture design for three cases

In order to demonstrate the principles, which have been described, to particular cases, three situations are considered, but it should not be inferred that these designs apply to all cases with similar teeth missing, as a variety of other factors may make the designs invalid.

Case 1 (Figure 10.19)

Stage I

Saddle (a) is a tooth-borne saddle, and (b) a tissue-borne saddle and these are, therefore, classified as such and outlined on the design sheet and on the study casts. Support from the teeth is obtained from occlusal rests positioned adjacent to the saddle (a) and mesial on the premolar tooth for saddle (b).

Stage II

Bracing arms are placed on the abutment teeth, above the survey lines. Movement is now restricted in a horizontal plane.

Stage III

The direct retainers are placed on the sides of the teeth as shown and the only movement now allowed for is one of rotation of the free-end saddle around the tips of the clasps. The rotation axes are shown and stability is obtained if rotation takes place about axis (y) by the occlusal rest on the premolar of

saddle (a). If rotation takes place about the axis (x), the direct clasp on the molar tooth of saddle (a) will provide stability. There is, therefore, little need for indirect retention but, if desired, and this may be so in an upper denture, it should be placed on the anterior teeth in the form of a plate since it is the furthest point anterior to the fulcrum axis.

Stage IV

It is now necessary to complete the design by connecting the parts together, and this is done by means of a lingual bar since it is a lower denture and indirect retention is deemed unnecessary. If indirect retention had been used, the connector would have been a modified continuous clasp – a dental bar.

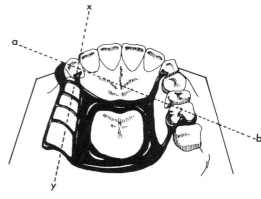

Figure 10.20 Case 2. Design of a unilateral free-end saddle denture

Case 2 (Figure 10.20)

In a unilateral saddle the stages I and II are similar to the single saddle (b) mentioned in the previous situation.

Stage III

Direct retention is provided on the abutment tooth, but this is quite inadequate and rotation may also take place along the saddle axes x–y. Stability and retention are, therefore, necessary, and the clasping unit is added to the molar tooth on the opposite side of the jaw, thus providing direct and indirect retention. This, however, provides a new fulcrum axis a–b and, in order to provide indirect retention, a Cummer rest is placed on the canine. This is very effective since it is as far from the fulcrum axis anteriorly as the applied load will be posteriorly.

Stage IV

Anterior and posterior palatal bars have been used since they can be fairly small in cross-section and unobtrusive to the tongue as large forces are not going to be developed in this situation. An alternative design would be a thin palatal plate covering the same area of the palate and this might be an advantage if retention on the free-end saddle were difficult to achieve on the canine tooth.

Case 3 (Figure 10.21)

A single anterior saddle is often a common problem in the upper jaw and the stages in developing a design are as follows.

Stage I

This is a bounded saddle and unless a decision has been made to use an Every design the rests are placed adjacent to the saddle on the two canines.

Stage II

Anteroposterior displacement is provided here by the rests and by the labial flange of the saddle. This is not enough; further stability must by provided by bracing arms on the premolar teeth which must be maintained in a stable position on the tooth by means of occlusal rests.

Stage III

Direct retention is difficult as the patient will object to clasps on the abutment teeth for aesthetic reasons. To be effective, retention must be as near the saddle as possible and would probably be placed on the premolar teeth. Apart from rotation of the saddle about the fulcrum axis when the saddle is pulled from the tissues, the denture would be stable, but to prevent rotation indirect retainers are thus placed on the molar teeth and in order to improve the retention, a complete clasping unit is provided.

Stage IV

To connect the parts together a horseshoe-type design is used since little force will be applied laterally in the posterior region.

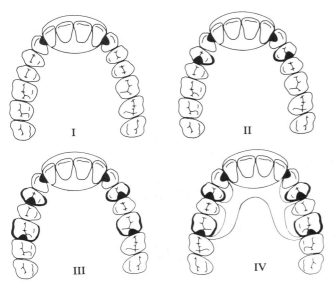

Figure 10.21 Case 3. Stages in the design of a denture with an anterior saddle only (Kennedy Class IV)

11

Mouth preparation

Following the design of the denture and the completion of the periodontal and surgical treatment, conservation of the teeth is commenced and their restoration must be carried out with the denture in mind. Where decayed teeth are concerned, a number of possible options exist.

Where the tooth is so badly broken down there are several courses of treatment. For instance, in an elderly patient where no root canal is visible on the radiograph, it may be necessary to extract the tooth. On the other hand, if this is a very important tooth, as an abutment, and in a relatively young patient, the decision to carry out endodontic treatment and restore the tooth with a full crown might be the ideal form of treatment. Alternatively, the endodontic treatment could be completed and a root face attachment fitted (Figure 11.1).

The tooth may require restoration, but not extensively, therefore the choice exists between a gold restoration or a plastic material. Ideally, in these circumstances, gold should always be used since it is much more resistant to flow and it is possible to carve the occlusal rest more satisfactorily in a restoration of this type without causing undue weakening of the restoration. Where possible, therefore, gold crowns would be the restoration of choice.

It is mandatory that any restoration must be constructed to the present or modified occlusion.

Full crowns as abutment restorations

The main advantages of using crowns, either anterior or posterior, are that all the ideal concepts which are discussed in the section concerning the preparations of the natural teeth can be easily included. Where aesthetics demand a porcelain bonded gold crown is used. Porcelain is hard enough to contour and use for clasping but, where possible, this should, and can usually, be avoided so that the retaining arm rests on a metal surface (Figure 11.2).

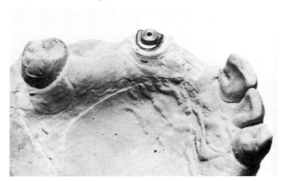

Figure 11.1 A root-faced attachment added to an endodontically treated tooth

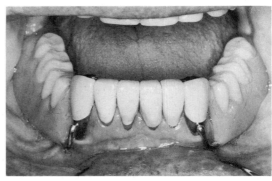

Figure 11.2 The retaining arms placed on the gold substructure rather than on the porcelain

Guiding planes

Since the paths of insertion and the design of the denture have already been determined before the tooth preparations are begun, it is easy to ensure that enough tooth structure is removed to enable the surfaces of the gold to be made parallel to the path of insertion of the denture in those areas adjacent to the saddles and on the lingual surfaces.

Provision of ledges for bracing and guiding planes

In Chapter 9 it was explained that the bracing arm and retaining arm should, where possible, be on the same horizontal plane and, in such circumstances, bracing and reciprocation are combined. Gold crowns allow this to be accomplished easily provided care is taken in preparing the tooth to allow for an adequate thickness of gold (Figure 11.3a). The arm

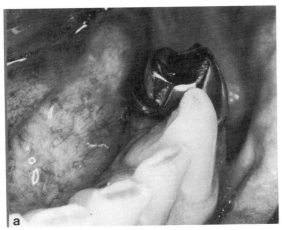

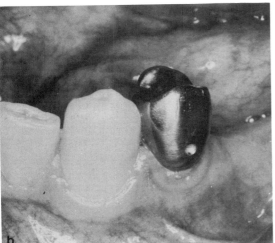

Figure 11.3 Gold crown prepared to allow for a recessed bracing arm and a gingivally approaching arm

thus provided is unobtrusive since it replaces the contour of the tooth and is preferable to the normal bracing arm which projects from the natural tooth surface, improving tolerance by the patient and, at the same time, increasing the guiding plane surface area. In many instances where enough guiding plane surfaces are used, direct retention can often be eliminated since the whole appliance is like a complicated precision attachment. Retention can, however, be easily obtained by using a gingivally approaching clasp arm fitted into a recess on the buccal side of the tooth (Figure 11.3b).

When the castings have been prepared and tried in the mouth they must be returned to the master cast which is then mounted on a surveyor or a milling machine and all the paths milled to form a single path of insertion. Finally, after polishing the restorations, the partial dentures can be constructed on the master cast, but it is preferable to cement the full crown in place and to retake the final impressions for partial denture construction.

The advantages are:

(1) The time required for the patient to wear temporary crowns is reduced with consequent improvement in gingival health and, in many cases, the dies on the master cast are not so rigidly held in place that some movement cannot take place during duplicating with consequent possible errors in the final casting.
(2) The final impression for crowns may not always be satisfactory for partial denture construction, particularly in free-end saddle cases where saddle extension may be inadequate.

Occlusal rest seats

Enough tooth structure should have been removed to enable the gold to be prepared for the rest seats as for the natural tooth. If enough tissue can be removed, it may be possible to prepare a steep box rest seat which can act not only as a rest, but also give some degree of bracing (Figure 11.4). This is not usually advocated, and if sufficient space exists in the tooth tissue, a precision attachment can usually be inserted.

Intracoronal restorations in abutment teeth

Gold inlays are not now commonly used, but may be for restorations of decayed teeth with mesial, distal and occlusal surfaces. Under these circumstances, the guiding planes can be arranged by contouring the inlay mesialy or distally to follow the path of insertion provided the tooth preparation has been carried out adequately. The occlusal rest seats can

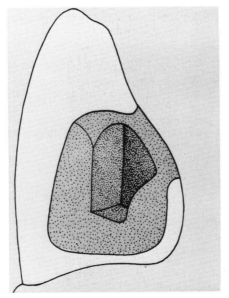

Figure 11.4 A steep-sided box rest seat which may be used to provide bracing as well as occlusal support

also be prepared in the gold in exactly the same way that they would be prepared in enamel.

Class V inlays may also be used to add contour to the tooth or, more usually, to have a depression cut into the surface into which a ball-ended gingival retainer is fitted (as in Figure 11.3), thus obtaining retention with minimum complexity. This type of clasp is particularly useful where no satisfactory undercuts exist in the natural tooth.

Preparation of the natural teeth prior to partial denture construction

The occlusion

If it has already been observed clinically, and with the mounted study casts, that the occlusion is in need of adjustment, then those modifications to the natural teeth must now be considered. The objectives of occlusal analysis have already been described in Chapter 1 and these must be achieved by occlusal grinding or the provision of crowns or the partial denture.

The techniques involved in occlusal correction have already been established and reference to the bibliography will give the reader a detailed description of the technique.

The use of a partial denture to provide an occlusion necessitates an overall view of the occlusion and to ignore the natural teeth whilst making a partial denture is failing to undertake the true task of the dentist which is to restore the patient's masticatory apparatus. Following any adjustment to the occlusion, it will be necessary to contour the natural teeth since they are seldom ideal for partial denture construction, but, as long as care is taken, there is no objection to grinding the enamel surface provided it is not excessive and the surface is adequately polished and then treated with a fluoride preparation.

Modification of the anterior teeth

Anterior support is gained by extension of the denture base on to the palatal, lingual and incisal surfaces of the teeth. These rests must not interfere with the natural occlusion or mastication, and must be smooth and non-irritating to the tongue as well as being concealed from view as much as possible.

Upper incisor teeth have natural inclines which offer very little direct rest support, but they can be made more effective by tooth preparation.

The first stage is the preparation of the proximal surface where there is a marked proximal curvature, as in posterior teeth, to provide guiding planes. The gingival part of the seat preparation should be as flat as possible and at right angles to the axis of the tooth, while the incisal segment should blend into the more vertical palatal tooth contour without sharp angulations which would tend to encourage accumulation of food debris and plaque. The marginal ridge at the junction of the proximal surface and the rest seat is reduced to increase the rest strength (Figure 11.5).

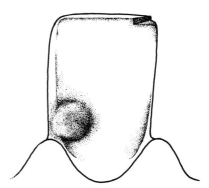

Figure 11.5 Rest seat preparation on an upper central incisor tooth

The palatal surface anatomy of canines is often characterized by a well-developed cingulum prominence which may be utilized for denture support and, with preparation, the support can be very positive. Extension on to the tooth surface adjacent to the edentulous saddle, in a similar way to the upper incisor tooth, is the most commonly used method, but in some instances the rest may be extended

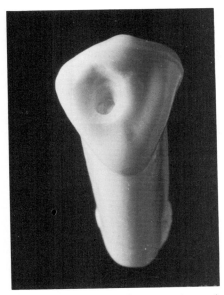

Figure 11.6 Preparation of a rest seat in a canine

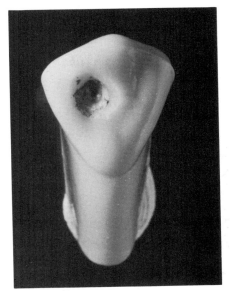

Figure 11.7 The rest seat finalized with the insertion of an amalgam filling

across the tooth. A simple method of preparing rest seats in canines is shown in Figure 11.6. A small round diamond is used to make a hole about 2 mm in diameter down to the level of the dentine–enamel junction. The cavity is then filled with amalgam which is left just short of the upper surface to create a depression. A ball-ended burnisher is used to compact the restoration (Figure 11.7).

The provision of adequate support on the lower anterior teeth is a much greater problem than in other segments of the mouth.

The mandibular anterior teeth have lingual surfaces which are steeper than the maxillary teeth; there is less cingulum development, less marginal ridge prominence and thinner enamel surfaces.

Lingual resting is, therefore, not very effective, even with limited tooth modification and an alternative method with an extension over the incisal margin of the lower abutment tooth, producing a rest with an axially directed force, is preferable (Figure 11.8).

Preparation of the tooth surface is essential to minimize an unfavourable aesthetic effect, and to

prevent interference to the occlusion, especially when a degree of attrition is present.

The stages in the preparation are similar to previous procedures and can be detailed as follows.

(1) Identify incisal contact areas for closure and function, with articulating paper.
(2) Determine the area of rest seat to be selected and prepare an incisal step of approximately 0.5 mm thickness and a horizontal seat floor.
(3) Prepare a slight labial bevel of approximately 0.5 mm and carry the bevel over the vertical wall of the step.
(4) Prepare a lingual bevel to the step, more extensively than labially (up to 1 mm) to give sufficient strength to the rest. The area is then smoothed and polished and treated with fluoride. The completed rest is seen to be unobtrusive from the labial view and blends into the lingual contours.

Mesial or distal incisal rests may be prepared dependent upon the type of adjacent saddle, and in some instances both incisal margins may carry a rest

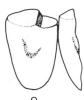 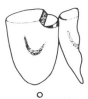 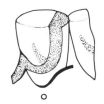

Figure 11.8 Incisal rest seats on lower incisor teeth. ○, lingual, ●, labial

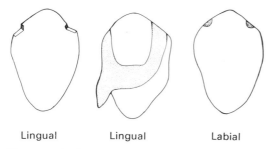

Lingual　　　Lingual　　　Labial

Figure 11.9 Incisal rest seats on a lower canine tooth

(Figure 11.9). The preparations are paralleled to the marginal contours and are more conservative in extent when compared with the single incisal rest preparation.

Another important step in the preparation of a mouth for partial dentures is the development of guiding plane inclines.

As the proximal surfaces of anterior teeth are mostly convex and some degree of tilting has usually occurred towards the edentulous spaces, construction of the denture saddles inevitably leads to some spacing between the seated denture and the natural teeth and these can be the sites for food impaction and areas that provide a very poor aesthetic appearance (Figure 11.10).

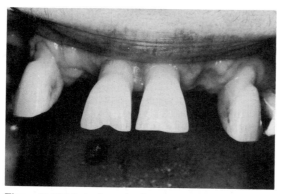

Figure 11.10 Marked proximal contours on anterior teeth which lead to spacers between the denture and the teeth giving a very poor aesthetic result

Ideally, all the proximal surfaces are paralleled, and the more of these planes that are distributed throughout the arch, the more restrictive and precise will be the path of insertion and withdrawal. This does not apply however for two part – sectional denture or swing lock dentures being constructed since the undercuts mentioned will be required for retention.

Because of the greater contact area between the appliance and the tooth surfaces, there is less potential for food impaction, and as the path of removal is more definite, retention is more effective.

Anterior abutment teeth frequently have heights of contour which present a problem in the aesthetic placement of retainers (Figure 11.11), but it is possible to modify the excessive contour on a labial or buccal surface by grinding and then polishing the surface.

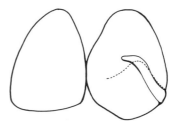

Figure 11.11 A survey line near the incisal edge on a canine tooth creates a retainer which is unaesthetic

The changed contour permits a retainer to be placed in a less visible position (Figure 11.12) or permits a tooth area to be used for retention where previously an excessive contour precluded this. This type of reduction is beneficial for gingivally approaching retainers also, rendering them less visible and less vulnerable to the cheek tissues.

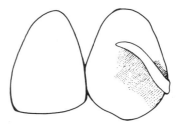

Figure 11.12 Adjustment of the tooth surface by grinding will enable the clasp to be placed more gingivally thus improving aesthetics

Tooth recontouring is advantageous where some drifting has taken place and difficulty is experienced in maintaining proportion between the artificial replacement and the natural dentition. Improved aesthetic effects can be obtained by recontouring the proximal surfaces of the standing teeth, but additional benefit can be derived by the irregular placement of the artificial teeth. Lapping of the natural teeth by the artificial, or placing the artificial teeth with less prominence than the natural teeth, are methods of creating the illusion of normal size in

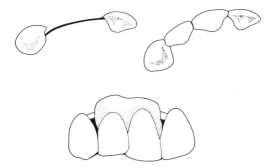

Figure 11.13 Cusped grooving to improve the placement of artificial anterior teeth

restricted areas. In Figure 11.13 cuspid grooving has been combined with labial discing of the incisor.

Modification of the posterior teeth

During functional movements vertical and oblique forces are directed by the occlusal rests on to the supporting structures where they are dissipated through the periodontal fibres to the underlying bone and these forces must not overload the periodontal fibres or damage to the tooth will arise.

Consideration of the denture design will disclose many areas where ideal conditions do not exist, and where modification of a tooth surface will improve the effectiveness of the occlusal rest.

Preparation will permit more direct force application to the tooth, will provide a rest that is less obtrusive to the tongue, and a rest which will not interfere with the opposing teeth when in occlusion. In some instances of tooth rotation, the rests may be palatally or lingually placed. Should most of the occlusal surface be involved in normal function, it is preferable to select an alternative site.

By virtue of the tooth form being tapered, as in premolars, there is a possibility that when a force is transmitted via an occlusal rest, a torque may develop on a tooth but this may be minimized by extension of the rest length towards the centre of the tooth, or by reduction of the curvature of the proximal surface (Figure 11.14).

The potential for a rotatory effect from the occlusal rests is increased if they are placed on tilted teeth. But again this may be minimized by angulation of the rest seat preparation to be in keeping with the tooth angulation, and reduction of the proximal surface contour to provide a guiding plane (Figure 11.15).

Despite the many variables involved, it is suggested that occlusal rests should have at least the following minimum dimensions – occlusal rest area 3 × 3 mm, occlusal rest thickness a minimum of 0.5 mm, and there should be a marginal ridge thickness of at least 1.5 mm.

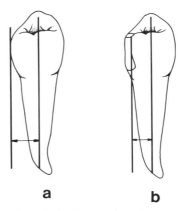

Figure 11.14 The torque produced by an occlusal rest in (a) can be reduced by grinding the proximal surface in (b)

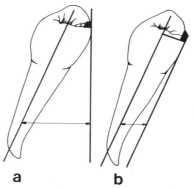

Figure 11.15 Torque on the tooth (a) may be minimized by angulation of the rest seat and the production of a guiding plane (b)

Tooth modification is also beneficial in conditions of marked attrition.

Where occlusal and incisal wear have developed the maximum contour of the abutment teeth frequently will be found to be at the occlusal surface or incisal margin itself.

The lack of an occlusal curvature above the height of contour complicates the insertion of the appliance for it is essential that a retainer be expanded by the tooth contour to allow it to slide into place (Figure 11.16). Without expansion the retainer arm will bind on the occlusal surface which should be planed with a diamond stone to replace normal surface contour. This also applies to some posterior teeth which are excessively tilted, such as lower third molars.

Even if sharp margins are not involved in retainer function, they should be modified, as sharp margins are difficult to reproduce on the working casts, and damage to them during the technical stages of construction will greatly complicate the insertion stage.

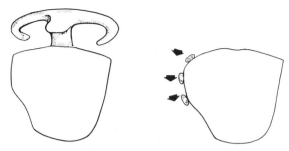

Figure 11.16 Occlusal grinding may be necessary to produce incline planes which will allow the clasp to flex into an undercut

Tooth modification is also beneficial for major connector placement. This is especially so where lingually inclined teeth complicate the design of the appliance.

When the teeth are inclined beyond the contours of the supporting soft tissues, and rigid connector bars or plates must pass them, extensive blocking out must result, with production of large food trapping areas.

Discing of the offending lingual contours will allow a more favourable placement of the denture components or, alternatively, if this is not possible a connector such as a buccal bar must be used (Figure 11.17).

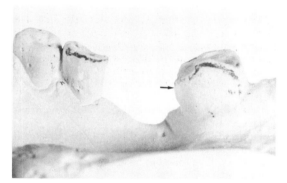

Figure 11.17 Excessively tilted teeth may lead to stagnation areas which could be improved by grinding the tooth surface

Tooth preparation divided into six stages

Stage I: the preparation of the proximal surface

The height of contour on the proximal surface is usually close to the occlusal surface with a convexity of the surface below, so that without preparation, the prosthesis could have only limited contact with the tooth surface. Reduction of the contour to a guiding plane or surface parallel to the path of

insertion would permit a more intimate contact between tooth and prosthesis. This will, in turn, produce a more positive seating action and provide less possibility for food impaction.

The surface is prepared using a diamond stone held parallel to the anticipated path of insertion (Figure 11.18).

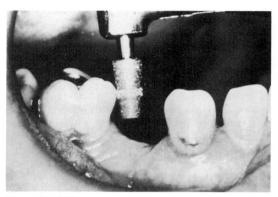

Figure 11.18 The use of a stone to prepare the guiding plane

Stage II: the preparation of the rest seat

The occlusal contacts are located by marking the closure with articulating paper and the area of the rest seat is determined. The preparation is then made using a 3 mm diameter round stone to produce a saucer-shaped depression (Figure 11.19).

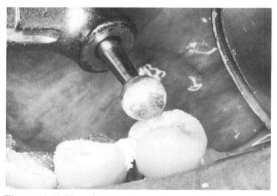

Figure 11.19 Use of a stone to produce a short saucer-shaped depression for the occlusal rest

Stage III: the marginal ridge preparation

As the greatest stress concentration in function will be at the junction of the rest and the connector, strengthening of the rest is assured by a reduction and rounding of the marginal ridge at the junction of the two previously prepared surfaces.

Stage IV

Fine carborundum stones are used to polish all ground surfaces, and they are followed by sand-paper discs and application of polishing pastes to give a smooth prepared surface.

Stage V

The rest area is dried and a suitable fluoride solution is applied to the ground areas.

Stage VI

An optional step, but recommended where heavy occlusal contact exists close to the rest area. A small piece of modelling wax is heated and adapted over the occlusal rest area and the patient is then encouraged to carry out lateral excursions and normal masticatory function. Subsequent examination of the wax will confirm whether or not the preparations that have been completed will allow adequate rest dimensions. With careful preparation the rest contours will restore normal anatomical contours to the tooth.

Rest preparation can be even more complicated, especially where the occlusal rest coverage is to be extended on to several adjacent teeth with multiple retaining arms (Figure 11.20). Here preparation is essential to allow rest placement which will not interfere with the occlusion and to provide contours to the teeth which will give sufficient strength to the clasp and avoid deformation or fracture. This may arise due to high buccal and palatal survey lines which necessitate thinning of the metal. Reduction of these areas is essential to lower the survey lines and give adequate strength to the rest and clasps (Figure 11.21).

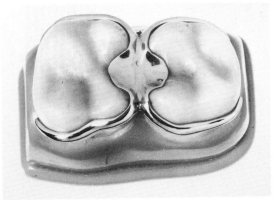

Figure 11.20 The occlusal rests on adjacent teeth with multiple retaining arms

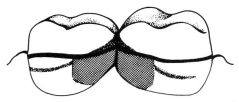

Figure 11.21 Grinding will lower the high survey lines and allow proper placement of the clasp arm

The marginal ridge preparation required is of a greater dimension than that for a simple rest, for the preparation must provide the space for an adequate connector for the two retainer arms. It is extended buccally and lingually to provide bulk for the retainers and the lingual minor connector.

12

Construction of partial dentures

Creating the impression

In order to construct a denture, it is necessary to have a master cast made which duplicates the mouth as accurately as possible. The details of the construction of a tray for a partial denture have already been described in Chapter 3, and final impressions for partial dentures usually taken in an irreversible hydrocolloid, such as alginate, or an elastomeric material, are described in Chapter 4, together with the casting of the impressions to form the master cast.

Preparation of the master cast

Tripod marks which are used to record the tilt of the cast on the surveyor and thus the path of insertion of the denture are described in Appendix IV and are shown in Figure 12.1.

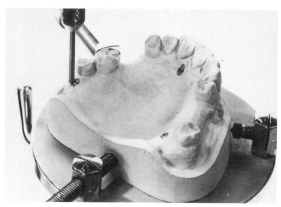

Figure 12.1 Marking three anatomical points on the cast in the same horizontal plane to form a tripod

These tripod marks are transferred to the master cast which can then be placed on the surveyor and the planned tilt already established during surveying of the study cast can be transferred to the master cast by arranging for the three tripod points to be in a perfectly horizontal plane. This is checked by fixing the height of the tip of the carbon rod in the surveyor making sure that it touches all three points. The master cast can now be surveyed (Figure 12.2).

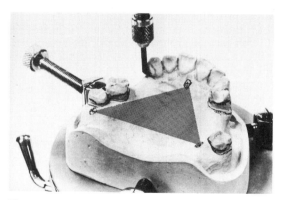

Figure 12.2 Surveying the master cast

The carbon rod is removed and replaced by an undercut gauge (Figure 12.3). Those teeth to which retentive arms are to be fitted are then selected by reference to the study casts and a second line drawn, below the survey line, with a 0.25 mm (0.10 inch) undercut in the region of the tip of the clasp. This line is produced by bringing the undercut gauge up to the tooth and noting the point at which the lateral part of the gauge touches the cast whilst the rod is in

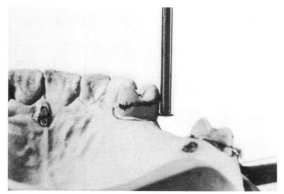

Figure 12.3 The use of an undercut gauge to ascertain the correct position of the tip of the clasp

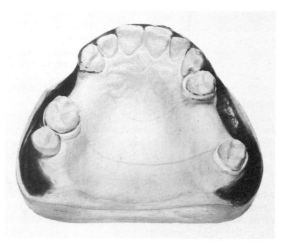

Figure 12.5 The undercuts blocked out with modelling wax

contact with the survey line. A line can now be drawn from the occlusal border of the clasp extending into the undercut area to a known depth (Figure 12.4).

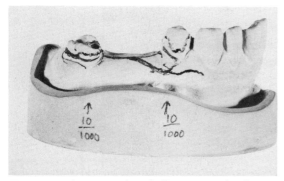

Figure 12.4 The preparation of a line representing the lower border of the clasp

Wax is then added to block out all undercuts except those used for retaining clasps. It is preferable to use special blocking-out wax on the teeth, but gross undercuts in a labial or buccal aspect of the cast, not involved with the denture construction, may be blocked out to excess with a good modelling wax (Figure 12.5).

Excess wax surrounding the teeth may be removed with a chisel placed in the surveyor (see Appendix IV.2). This is a most important stage in the partial denture construction, as any excess wax occlusal to the survey line means that the guiding planes are lost and if excess trimming with the chisel results in rubbing away of the stone cast, the saddle area will be too large to fit between the teeth. For this reason, a stone cast with a high abrasive resistance is required.

All soft tissue undercuts should also be eliminated by the use of modelling wax and, if a plate covering

the teeth is used, the interproximal spaces between the teeth must also be filled in with wax. In the upper the outlines of the palatal connectors (food lines) are scraped on the cast with a sharp tool to a depth of about 0.5–1 mm. The edges of these grooves should be slightly rounded, and when the casting is complete, these grooves are reproduced as raised borders on the fitting surfaces of the appliance. These ridges apply a slight pressure to the tissues and prevent food and saliva from passing under the connectors which can be unpleasant for the patient. For this reason the grooves on the master cast are sometimes termed 'food lines'.

On those teeth where the clasps are to be fitted, wax is added to block out all the undercut below the level of the clasp arm. Excess wax may be added to form a shelf at the lower border of a clasp arm to act as a means of positioning the preformed pattern on the refactory cast (Figure 12.6). When a lingual bar

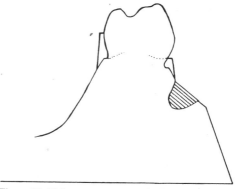

Figure 12.6 Master cast prepared with ledgers on the sides of the teeth to enable the preformed patterns to be correctly positioned on the investment cast

is to be used in the lower jaw, a similar ledge may be built on the master cast to help to position the wax pattern.

Applying relief

In many situations it is necessary to apply a thin relief over gingival margins, alveolar tissues, and over saddles to keep the metal away from the tissues.

Relief is usually provided over the saddle area where the metal part of the denture will be constructed. This is done in order that the acrylic resin saddle will then flow under the metal and cover the entire saddle area. Subsequent resorption of the tissues may necessitate a reline of the saddle and this can then be carried out more simply than if the base is in metal. Also, if the denture base requires easing after fitting, it is much easier to grind and polish the acrylic resin than it would be if it had been constructed in metal. In free-end saddles the relief on the master cast in this area is usually made of soft metal or wax (0.5–0.7 mm) and generally a small area, 2–3 mm square, is cut out of the material on the crest of the ridge so that when the casting is made it can be positioned on the master cast in its correct relationship.

It is common practice also to relieve (0.1 mm) all gingival margins over which clasp arms or minor connectors need to cross. Palatal bars and lingual bars may also need relief if it is anticipated that the connector may sink into the tissues and cause trauma. This particularly applies in areas like the midline of the palate and the lingual surfaces of the alveolus in the lower premolar regions where the mucosal tissues are relatively thin.

Duplication of the master cast

The prepared master cast is now ready to be duplicated. The cast is soaked in warm water (40°C) for 20 minutes to fill all the 'pores' of the stone and displace trapped air. While this is taking place the agar-agar duplicating material may be heated in a double boiler to 95°C when it will become quite fluid. The inner pan is then removed and the agar should be stirred and allowed to cool slowly until it reaches approximately 52°C depending on the manufacturer's instructions. These materials exhibit hysteresis, that is, the temperature at which they change from a gel to a sol is higher than when they pass from a sol to a gel state. If large numbers of castings are to be made in a laboratory it is preferable to use a large bath kept at the correct

temperature for pouring, since this eliminates time wasted in heating up the agar for individual casts.

Provided that the base of the cast is flat, it will sit on the base of the duplicating flask without sealing (Figure 12.7), but if in doubt it may be held in place by Plasticine. Remove excess water from the surface

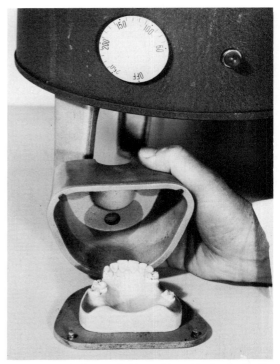

Figure 12.7 Master cast being positioned in the duplicating flask

of the cast and run the agar-agar carefully into a hole in the upper part of the flask. These holes are usually positioned in the corners of the flask and the agar therefore flows on to a corner of the cast (Figure 12.8). Allow to cool for 30 minutes and then place in a bath of running tap water, about 2.5 cm deep for about 20 minutes. When adequately gelled, remove the base of the flask and cut two pieces of agar away from the sides of the cast to allow the base to be gripped with the fingers (Figure 12.9). If difficulty is experienced, the mould may be removed from the duplicating flask and the cast removed gently. Provided the agar mould is then restored to a duplicating flask, no dimensional error should result. The refractory material should have been weighed or measured out while the agar-agar material was cooling and it can then be rapidly mixed and poured into the mould as soon as the master cast is removed.

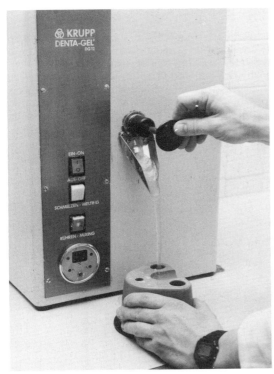

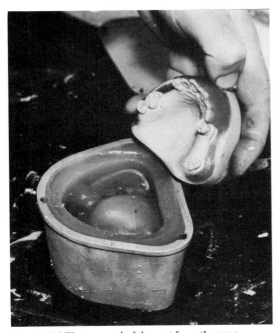

Figure 12.8 Duplicating material running into the flask

Figure 12.9 The removal of the cast from the agar duplicating material

Pouring the investment cast

The majority of modern techniques use an investment of phosphate-bonded silica. Usually about 200 g of investment with the requisite amount of water (about 12 ml per 100 g), or in some cases a water solution made up with a special silica fluid, is needed for each cast.

The investment may set rapidly with the production of a large exotherm and it is therefore necessary to vibrate the powder into the water and to mix with a mechanical spatula under vacuum as rapidly as possible (Figure 12.10). Mixing should be complete between 30 and 60 seconds. The duplicating flask with the mould is placed on the vibrator and the slurry run down one side until the deepest part of

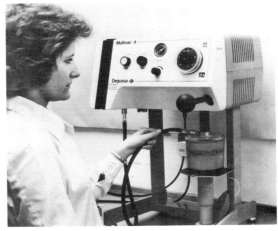

Figure 12.10 Investment material mixed with a mechanical spatula under vacuum

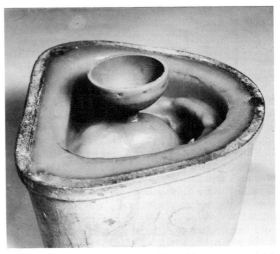

Figure 12.11 A sprue former positioned in the agar mould

the mould is filled. Investment is then moved around the mould using the vibrator to ensure that no air is trapped. The rest of the cast can then be poured rapidly, slightly underfilling the mould. In some instances, where sprues will eventually pass through the base of the cast, a sprue former may be used to ensure that a hole is provided (Figure 12.11). Many technicians, however, prefer to drill a hole in the cast after the investment has set.

After about 1 hour the agar-agar mould is removed from the flask and taken from the refractory cast in small pieces to prevent damage to the investment which is very friable at this stage (Figure 12.12).

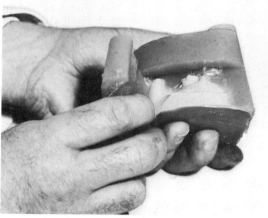

Figure 12.12 Removal of the agar duplicating material in small pieces from the refractory cast

Hardening the cast

The cast should be trimmed down to its minimum size, sloping the edges to make the base smaller than the periphery of the cast. If a model trimmer is used, the cast should be cut dry and the machine flushed with water when completed. This helps to ensure adequate retention to the embedding investment at a later stage. It is then dried in an oven at 100°C for 2 hours and when dry it can be either sprayed with a proprietary aerosol material or dipped in molten hardening wax. This can be a dangerous procedure and care must be taken to see that the model is dry and the beeswax and resin mixture melted in a thermostatically controlled electric bath. These materials are absorbed into the cast and when cold provide a hard surface which prevents the invest-ment from being rubbed away. The dipping wax should be melted at 130°C and the cast immersed until frothing ceases. The cast is then removed and allowed to drain so that excess wax does not remain on the surface.

The wax pattern

The wax pattern of the partial denture is formed on the hardened investment cast and it is usual to use preformed wax or plastic shapes (Figure 12.13), which are glued into place. The parts of the pattern can be constructed by free-hand waxing, but this is more time-consuming and it is unlikely that the dimensions of the parts will be as consistent as when preformed patterns are used.

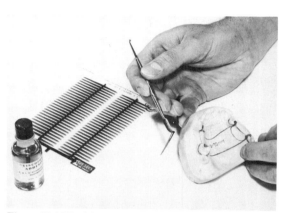

Figure 12.13 Positioning the preformed clasp patterns on the investment cast

Partial dentures vary in design so much that it would be impossible to cover all the possible designs and therefore only a broad outline of the essential points which help to produce a good wax pattern can be covered in this chapter. Where possible, the waxes selected should be of such a colour that they contrast with the colour of the investment cast since this reduces the fatigue of the operator in laying down these patterns. A further point which should be emphasized is that care spent in producing a wax pattern is very well rewarded, by reducing the necessary time in finishing the denture, and ensures that bars, etc. are of the correct dimension. It is essential that the operator conducts the procedure with neatness and cleanliness. Where occlusal on-lays are required, it may be necessary to mount the refactory cast in centric relation to the opposing cast in order to obtain the correct occlusion in the wax.

The mandibular denture

The outline of the denture should be quite clear on the cast, but if it is not it should be pencilled in carefully with a soft lead pencil before starting to put down the pattern.

The procedure for producing a wax pattern should be consistent for all cases as this reduces the possibility of errors. It is suggested that the first part to be laid down should be the connectors and in the case of a lower denture, the lingual connector is the first important segment. The limit of the lower border of the connector, relative to the floor of the mouth and the gingival tissues, should be clearly defined since any impingement on the soft tissues of the mouth will ultimately lead to damage. As a guide, it is usual to allow 2–3 mm space between the gingivae and the connector on the upper surface and at least 1 or 2 mm from the soft tissues on the lower surface. A ledge may have been produced on the master cast and this simplifies this stage in the production of the wax pattern.

The lingual bar is produced from a shaped rod of wax about 1.5 mm thick (Ruscher's No.4). When a long span is being constructed it may be necessary to add wax to the lower edge to increase the rigidity of the bar, making it 'pear-shaped' (Figure 12.14).

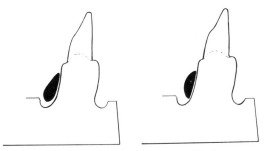

Figure 12.14 Pear-shaped lingual bar used for long connectors and the preformed shape for short spans

A plate is constructed from a 0.6 or 0.7 mm sheet of casting wax, placed from the lower border to the gingival margins from saddle to saddle. Then a 0.5 mm sheet of wax is laid over the entire lingual surface of the teeth, depending on the length of the structure. With a sharp knife, the wax is trimmed to the correct outline (Figure 12.15) and sealed down with a hot knife.

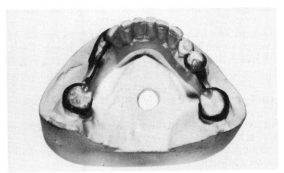

Figure 12.15 The completed wax pattern with lingual plate sealed down to the cast with a hot wax knife

A modified Kennedy continuous clasp or dental bar may be used and the wax pattern is prepared by laying down two sheets of 0.5 mm wax plus additions of fluid wax to make the thinnest portion over the cingulums at least 1.0 mm.

Sublingual bars are best constructed by placing a normal wax pattern round side down on the cast and adding wax to give the necessary contour. Buccal bars, because of their extra length, are more flexible and need to be thicker than normal lingual bars.

The next stage is to produce a saddle which will eventually retain the acrylic resin parts of the denture. Several methods are used to retain the acrylic which vary from a mesh to loops of wax joined to a central bar (Figure 12.16). The hole in the relief for free-end saddles must be filled in with wax before the pattern is laid. The wax saddle should extend to about two-thirds the length of the ridge and if no step has been provided in the relief it should pass just distal to the relief area so that it touches on to the unrelieved parts of the cast. The junction with the connector should be such that the connector is thicker than the saddle and the step thus provided can be used for finishing the acrylic resin flush with the metal (Figure 12.15 and 12.16).

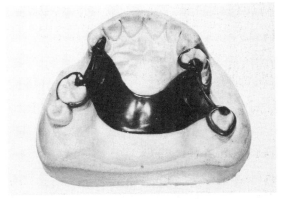

Figure 12.16 Junction of the saddle and the connector provided with a finishing edge for the acrylic resin

The minor connectors are made of semi-circular wax rods 1.5 mm wide (Ruscher's No.6) and are sealed to the saddles and adapted to the guiding planes of the abutment teeth and finally bent over the occlusal surface to form the occlusal rests. Wax is added freehand and the rest carved to shape. It is most important that the wax pattern should be sealed to the cast at the edges or investment will run underneath the wax pattern when the cast and pattern are finally embedded.

The preformed clasp pattern is selected and the cast painted with glue and then starting at the tip and working back to the junction with the minor connector the pattern is placed in position. The excess pattern is cut off and the junction of the minor connector and the clasp sealed with molten wax by a free-hand waxing method. The pattern is now completed and should be examined carefully to see that all the junctions of the parts are smooth and continuous. Where parts meet at right angles the junction should be rounded rather than finished at sharp angles. The pattern should not be flamed but smoothed by carving.

The maxillary denture

Where food lines are present the outline of the denture will be quite clear, but in other areas this should be pencilled in lightly as for the lower denture. The first stage is to produce, as in the lower denture, the connecting bars or plates and these are usually prepared by laying down a 0.5 mm sheet of casting wax over the palate to form a plate or connecting bar. If a plate is to be used, similar to that in Figure 12.17, it is possible to use wax with a stippled surface to simulate the palatal tissues. Most manufacturers of preformed patterns make a wax of this type or, alternatively, there are techniques for reproducing the actual mucosal surfaces of the patient for this type of pattern. It has merit in so far that the irregularities of the surface tend to increase the rigidity of the structure but do collect stain and can be difficult to keep clean.

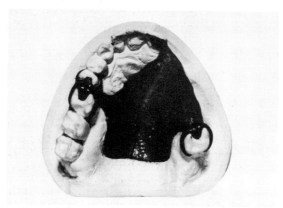

Figure 12.17 The use of a stippled wax to simulate palatal tissues

When the palate is deep it is often preferable to use two sheets of wax and join them in the middle to prevent thinning of the pattern when it is pressed into place. Where bars are used it is preferable to thicken them by the addition of a second sheet of wax of 0.5–0.7 mm and then cutting out the bars to the food lines (Figure 12.18). With a hot knife the two waxes are sealed to the cast and polished. If the palate is wide and there is no anterior palatal bar the posterior one should be thickened.

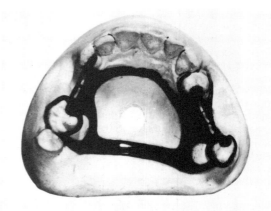

Figure 12.18 The finished upper wax pattern with anterior and posterior palatal bars

The order for preparing retention for the acrylic resin saddle and the rests, etc. is similar to that for the lower denture. A finishing line is placed along the edge of the saddle to demarcate the extent of the acrylic resin and the palatal connectors (Figure 12.16).

If the denture includes an anterior tooth it may be necessary to make a palatal surface for the tooth in metal and add the tooth as a facing. The wax pattern is prepared after positioning the tooth and checking the occlusion with a lower cast, to ensure that it will not cause interference when the casting is complete. Occasionally, an all-metal saddle will be required for a posterior tooth, but this is not usual practice and unless there is a specific reason it is unnecessarily time-consuming to produce and a disadvantage from the technical point of view.

The preparation of the clasps, etc. is in every way similar to the lower pattern.

Sprueing

Once the pattern has been completed it is necessary to provide some means whereby the metal can flow in from the outside of the mould into the cavity formed when the wax pattern is eliminated. These entrances are usually provided by wax rods called sprues which are joined to the pattern and run to the crucible former. The positioning of the sprues needs great care as failure to place them correctly means that the mould may not fill with metal and all the labour of the construction of the partial denture is wasted.

There are two ways of sprueing a pattern; either from above (Figure 12.19) called 'top sprueing', or from below, called 'inverted sprueing' (Figure 12.20). For a metal which is viscous and where the

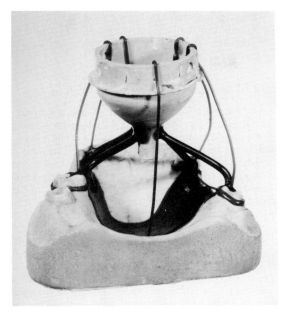

Figure 12.19 A wax pattern sprued from above. The fine wax rods (air vents) allow the air to escape from the mould as the metal is forced in through the thicker sprues

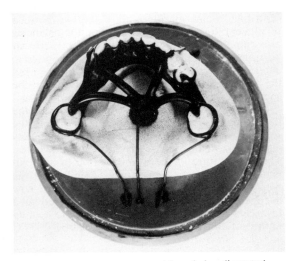

Figure 12.20 Wax pattern sprued from below (inverted sprueing)

cast is not very porous, air vents are often used. These are fine wax threads run from the junction of the sprue and the casting to the outer part of the mould. These allow trapped air to escape which would otherwise accumulate in the mould and prevent the proper ingress of metal. Partial dentures are always cast by multiple sprues which should be

so arranged that the metal flows in a continuous stream into the casting without being interrupted by sharp angles which will cause turbulence in the metal and also erode the investment leading to inaccuracies. The following points regarding sprues apply to whichever method of sprueing is adopted:

(1) The sprues should be large enough to allow the molten metal in them to remain liquid until the denture base has frozen.
(2) The sprues should pass into the mould cavity as directly as possible and still permit a configuration which will induce the minimum amount of turbulence in the stream of molten metal. 'Cast cracking' of the plate is prevented by curved sprues. As the metal contracts the radius of curvature of the sprue is increased and crushes the investment. With straight sprues this is not possible and the stress may cause fracture of the plate.
(3) Sprues should leave the crucible from a common point and be attached to the pattern at its bulkier sections; that is, no thin sections of casting should intervene between two bulky unsprued portions.

In many cases reservoirs are added to the area of the sprue just before its attachment to the wax pattern. The reservoirs are usually about three times as thick as the sprue. These large masses of metal remain molten for a considerable time and allow the casting to shrink as it cools and still draw liquid metal from the reservoir to replace metal 'lost' due to contraction.

The casting process

When the wax pattern has been sprued it is necessary to embed the whole cast and wax pattern in an investment similar to the cast itself. This outer investment should be at least 6 mm thick in its thinnest part and is confined around the cast by placing a ring around the pattern. The plastic ring is removed after the setting of the investment.

The investment particles must be of varying sizes in order that they pack on to the wax pattern, thus giving a smooth surface to the metal casting. The investment must also be porous enough to let air out as the metal enters the mould, or air vents should be added.

The sprued cast is sealed to the base of the ring. If top sprueing is used the crucible former should be level with the upper part of the ring. The wax pattern may be painted with a detergent solution (2% Teepol or Lisapol) which reduces surface tension and allows the investment to coat the wax surface without the formation of bubbles.

Investing the wax pattern

The investment should be mixed in the same way as the investment cast and in accordance with the manufacturer's instructions. If possible, it is best mixed with a power mixer under vacuum, as this eliminates nearly all the trapped air and enables the investment to be vibrated into the ring with little fear of air-bubbles being trapped on the wax pattern (Figure 12.21).

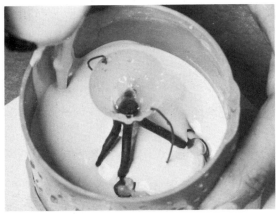

Figure 12.21 The ring is filled with investment material produced by mixing under a vacuum

If vacuum equipment is not available, mix the investment in a rubber bowl, as for plaster of Paris, and then paint the investment on to the pattern with a camel-hair brush, pushing it about until an even coat is applied and making sure no air-bubbles are trapped on the wax pattern (Figure 12.22).

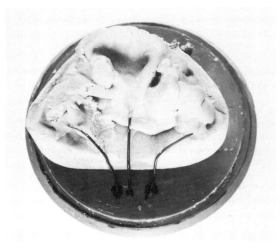

Figure 12.22 Investment brushed onto the wax pattern

When the investment has set, the ring is removed and the ends of the investment smoothed parallel to one another by rubbing the surface on coarse sandpaper.

The heating cycle

In the 'lost-wax process' used for all dental castings, it is necessary to eliminate the wax by slow heating of the investment. When the bulk of the wax is eliminated in an oven the ring is transferred to a furnace and the temperature raised slowly and sufficiently to give the necessary thermal expansion of the investment, thereby increasing the size of the mould cavity. In many industrial processes the molten metal is poured into the mould cavity by gravitational force which is sufficient, but in dental casting the alloy is not very fluid and the intricacy of the pattern necessitates a greater force than that created by gravity. This increased force can be applied by compressed air, steam or by the use of a centrifuge. The former methods were used for gold castings, but for the base metal alloys a centrifuge is always essential. In order to ensure that adequate centrifugal force is produced and at the same time prevent damage to the machine, the weight of the casting ring and the arm of the centrifuge must be balanced by a weight on the opposing arm of the centrifuge. Some machines allow the two arms to pivot from the centre. The weight on the balancing arm can then be adjusted until the are perfectly horizontal. In some machines, the ring size is used to determine the position of the counter weights, but the general principles of most machines are the same.

When the casting machine has been balanced, the rings may be placed in a preheating oven with the sprues pointing downwards, thus preventing any pieces of loose material falling into the sprue holes. The temperature of the oven is raised to approximately 300°C over 1–1½ hours, depending on the type of investment used. The wax will have now been eliminated and the ring is transferred to a furnace which is automatically controlled to heat up to the required casting temperature of about 1050°C in 1–1½ hours.

Casting techniques

The cobalt–chromium alloys have a melting range of 1200–1300°C and it is necessary to use electrical induction melting.

Induction melting

Many induction machines are available, but the Galoni machine (shown in Figure 12.23) and the Krupp machine are typical of the kind used for this

currents which generate considerable heat in an alloy which has a high electrical resistance. The cooling of the coil is essential to prevent it melting itself in the process. If an alloy which is a good electrical conductor, such as gold, is used the heating effect is much slower and it is essential to use a carbon-lined crucible to speed up the process and also to help reduce oxidation.

The carriage is positioned over the coil which is then raised around the crucible. The alloy is placed in the crucible and the machine is switched on.

The heating control is pressed and, as this is being done, the ring is placed in position and the heating completed. The molten alloy should only be observed through a blue glass screen. When the alloy is molten the coil is moved downwards away from the crucible (Figure 12.25) which allows the carriage to move up to the ring, and at the same time the motor is started to drive the centrifuge. When the casting is completed, the ring may be removed and allowed to cool.

Removing the investment from the casting

The cobalt–chromium alloys are not very susceptible to heat treatment and provided the ring is left to cool for 30 minutes optimum mechanical properties will result. The investment is removed by tapping the button of the casting with a hammer (Figure 12.26). The outer coating of the casting will have a considerable amount of chromium oxide attached to it. This, together with the remaining investment, is difficult to remove and a grit or shot-blaster is necessary. Sand is projected by compressed air through a fine nozzle on to the casting and these high-speed silica particles abrade the surface of the

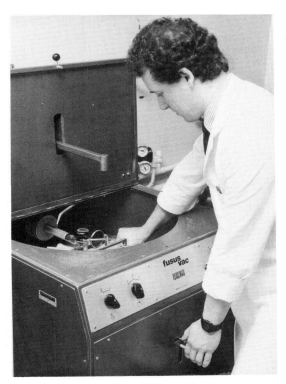

Figure 12.23 The Galloni casting machine

purpose. The electric motor drives the centrifuge, whilst a high frequency current which passes through a water-cooled coil is used to melt the alloy (Figure 12.24). The high-frequency current generates an alternating magnetic field in the alloy in a manner similar to the core of a solenoid. These high-frequency alternating fields produce induced

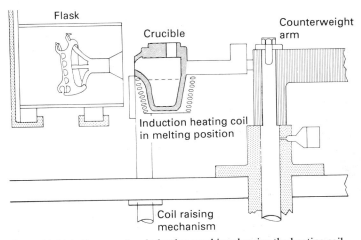

Figure 12.24 A diagram of an induction machine showing the heating coil

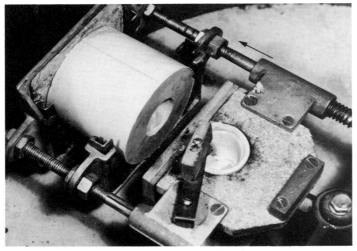

Figure 12.25 When the alloy is molten the coil is moved downwards from the crucible and the crucible slides forward to contact the casting ring

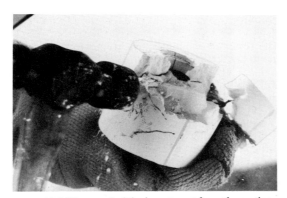

Figure 12.26 Removal of the investment from the casting

casting and break away any remaining debris (Figure 12.27). Once the casting is satisfactorily cleaned, the sprues may be removed.

Removal of the sprues

When removing the sprues a cut-off disc in a high-speed lathe (Figure 12.28) is used. It is essential that the operator wears a protective face-shield in case the cut-off disc shatters during the process. Great care must be taken at this stage to prevent any warpage of the casting caused by applying undue pressure to the sprues or the casting. Once the casting has been freed from the sprues it is usual to trim the surfaces roughly where the sprues have been, either on a high-speed wheel or using a

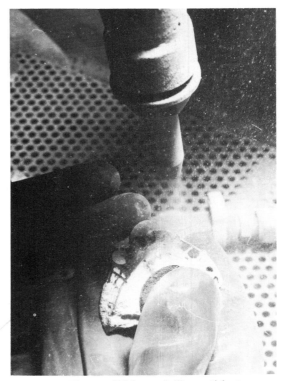

Figure 12.27 The use of high speed silica particles to remove the investment from the casting

stone in a dental handpiece. Rough edges on the clasps or parts of the denture may be ground to give a reasonably smooth surface (Figure 12.29).

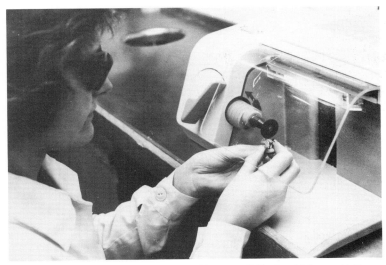

Figure 12.28 The removal of the sprues with a cut-off disc in a high speed lathe

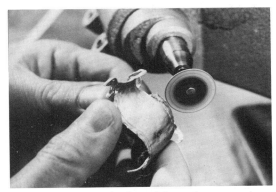

Figure 12.29 The rough edges of the casting removed

The addition of wrought clasps

If wrought clasps are to be added to the casting it is better to do it at this stage before further polishing. If stainless-steel clasps are used, they must be retained in the denture by being embedded in the acrylic resin of the saddles since soldering reduces the corrosion resistance of stainless steel. The more common types of wrought wires used are the platinized gold alloy wire of a minimum of 1 mm in diameter or a similar wire of nickel–chromium composition. The position of the wire clasps should have already been prepared in the actual casting by providing the necessary groove in the wax pattern during the waxing-up stage. All that needs to be done now is to bend the clasp approximately to shape on the tooth, leaving an excess of wire at the attaching end. The denture and clasp should be cleaned thoroughly and the clasp placed in position in the groove provided.

Soldering with the microwelder

It has been shown that gold can be soldered to base metal alloys satisfactorily. The best technique is to place the gold wire in position, using the very fine oxygen/hydrogen flame produced from the micro-welder (Figure 12.30). The two parts to be soldered are coated with a flux, which is allowed to dry, and the solder is then applied to the joint which, when heated, will draw the molten solder into the hottest part of the flame and surround the wires being soldered.

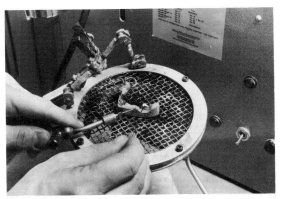

Figure 12.30 Soldering with a microwelder

Solders

Two types of solder are used in the soldering of cobalt–chromium alloys. For nickel–chromium wires a white alloy solder is used and, for the gold wires, a gold solder with a melting point 50°C less than the melting point of the wire is used. The composition of these solders can be obtained from a text on dental materials.

The essential points about a solder are as follows:

(1) It must have a melting point below that of the parts being joined, but as near to them as possible to make the strongest possible joint. The difference in the melting points of cobalt–chromium–nickel solders is quite large and the solder is relatively soft.
(2) It must have a low surface tension when molten.
(3) It should be of pleasing colour and be corrosion resistant.
(4) It should have adequate mechanical properties to withstand the forces to which the structure is subjected.

Fluxes

The fluxes used for soldering cobalt–chromium alloys are usually proprietary ones, but it is generally accepted that their principal constituents are potassium fluoride and borax. These proprietary materials fulfil the requirements of a flux in not efflorescing and flowing freely over the parts at a lower melting point than the solder. To be successful they must be good at dissolving the metallic oxides from the surface of the metal and in alloys composed of cobalt–chromium where the excellent corrosion resistance depends on an automatic self-sealing oxide layer; this is a difficult task and accounts for the problems when soldering these metals.

Once the soldering is complete, the denture is cleaned of any flux and the soldered areas stoned down to the final shape. The casting is then returned to the master cast for final shaping of the clasp. The mechanical properties of the base metal wires depend upon cold working and therefore this final bending completes the clasp. Where gold platinized wires are used, heat treatment may be required to obtain the optimum mechanical properties, but if a highly platinized wire is used, this is not usually necessary.

Polishing

Electrolytic

In this type of equipment, the casting acts as the anode of an electrolytic bath where the cathode is usually stainless steel. The electrolyte may be of

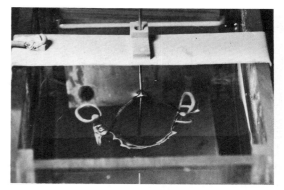

Figure 12.31 The denture attached to the anode of a polishing bath

several different types, but the one most commonly employed in the dental field is one based on phosphoric acid and glycerine.

The denture is attached and lowered into the electrolytic bath, as shown in Figure 12.31, and the current through the cell is raised to approximately 3 A at 6 V. The time taken to polish the denture depends upon the temperature of the solution and, if possible, it is preferable to keep the solution slightly warm in order to speed up the reaction. It is usual to give the casting 5 minutes in the bath and then to remove and wash it before replacing it in the bath for a further 5 minutes. The solution becomes quite warm at the end of the process and care must be taken to ensure that over-polishing does not reduce the size of clasps, etc. unnecessarily.

In order to prevent the fit of the denture from being destroyed, the inner aspect of clasps should be protected by either a wax coating or by painting with a mixture of shellac and methylated spirit, coloured by a little dye from an indelible pencil. This purple solution can be coated quite easily on to the inner side of the clasp which will then not be attacked by the electrolytic process. When the denture has reached this stage, it may be seated on the master cast and then tried in the patient's mouth to assess the fit before proceeding with what is always a laborious task, the final polishing. At this stage the surface will be uneven but shiny and the tissue surface should need little attention. In most cases, the denture can now be mechanically smoothed (Figure 12.32).

Mechanical

The first stage of mechanical polishing is with a rubber wheel impregnated with an abrasive agent which will impart to the surface of the casting a fairly high polish, as shown in Figure 12.33. The whole of the non-fitting surface is covered in this way to obtain a bright mirror-like surface. The second stage

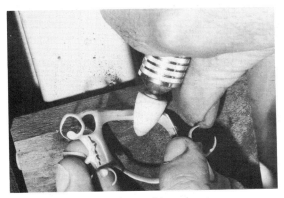

Figure 12.32 Mechanical smoothing using stones

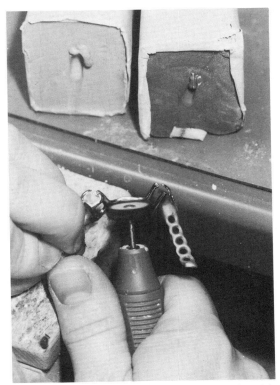

Figure 12.34 The use of a proprietary compound on a felt wheel for final polishing

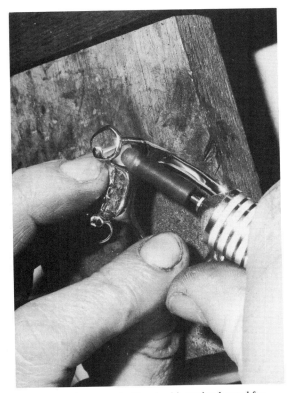

Figure 12.33 Impregnated hard rubber wheels used for polishing

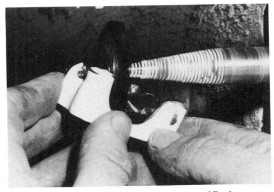

Figure 12.35 A denture backed by plaster of Paris to prevent damage from polishing on a dental lathe

is to polish the surface using a felt wheel or bristle brush in a handpiece and a proprietary polishing block to obtain a still finer surface (Figure 12.34). In some cases, specially impregnated felt wheels may be used to finalize and obtain a bright surface and they are of particular advantage on intricate surfaces. If desired, an ordinary dental lathe, using a brush and polishing paste, may also be used, but care must be taken to ensure that clasps are not bent in the process as they easily catch in the brush and it is worth while making a plaster cast to back up the casting during this polishing process (Figure 12.35). The denture can be finally cleaned in an ultrasonic bath to remove grease and dirt, or washed in a detergent solution. The blocking-out wax and reliefs are removed from the cast and the denture seated on it to ensure that it is a perfect fit.

Free-end saddle situations

In Chapter 10 the problem of the free-end saddle was discussed and special impression techniques were suggested (see p. 66) to obtain more support for the denture and to prevent rocking of the denture during mastication. One such technique is to tin-foil the master cast over the free-end saddle area or to use an alginate separating material and add a self-polymerizing acrylic resin saddle to the denture which, when set, is trimmed and polished to the normal saddle shape. The denture is then ready for the clinical stage of recording the occlusion.

13

Trials for metal and acrylic resin partial dentures

Metal partial dentures

Now that the casting has been completed, the next stage is to ensure that it fits accurately in the patient's mouth. The parts of the denture should fit as planned with no rocking about the occlusal rests. In the case of bilateral free-end saddle dentures, this is sometimes difficult to assess as the denture may rotate on only two occlusal rests, and in order to prevent this the addition of indirect retainers to the design may be useful as four rests would then be available to stabilize the denture. Alternatively, the technician may add a strut from the centre of the lingual bar to the incisal edges of the teeth. This can then be removed once the correcting impression is taken. Korrecta wax is used for impression taking and the clinical details are described by Applegate (1965).

Once the impression has been taken the denture is returned to the laboratory where the saddle area of the master cast is cut away, the denture reseated on the cast, and the periphery boxed in with wax on the lingual side (Figure 13.1). The cast is soaked in water for 10 minutes and new stone is poured into the impression to complete the master cast. The self-polymerizing acrylic resin saddle is removed and replaced by a wax saddle and occlusal rim and the denture returned to the clinic/surgery for the occlusion to be recorded.

Recording centric occlusion

The wax occlusal rims should be trimmed in the clinic until it is possible to establish a slight space between the teeth and the wax occlusal rims when the natural teeth are in centric occlusion. The occlusion of the natural teeth is checked and if

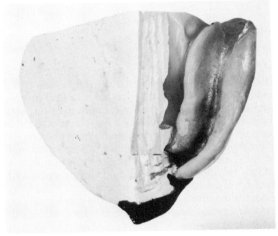

Figure 13.1 The removal of the saddle area from the master cast, placement of partial denture and boxing in on the lingual side

unsatisfactory either the denture or the natural teeth are ground until the teeth are in their normal centric occlusion.

If the centric occlusion of the natural teeth does not coincide with the centric jaw relation this should have been discovered at an early stage and corrected, or will be corrected by the partial denture. At this stage, therefore, there should be no difficulty in deciding on the centric occlusion that is to be recorded.

The technique for recording jaw relations with partial dentures is described in detail by Beckett (1954), who divides the possible situations into four categories as follows.

Type A

There is sufficient occlusal contact to render the relation of the upper and lower casts so obvious that no occlusal rims are required.

Type B

If there is insufficient occlusal contact to permit placing the casts in a definite relationship, then a definite relationship can be established by using an occlusal rim supported in the Class I and Class III saddle area by means of occlusal rests or other support on the teeth.

Type C

There is occlusal contact between some opposing teeth and/or Class I or III saddles to act as a stop for the purpose of establishing the correct vertical dimension. But this occlusal surface is not sufficient to permit placing the cast in the correct centric relation and, in addition, there are one or more Class II saddles which must also be used to establish centric and other relations.

Type D

There is no occlusal contact between opposing teeth and/or Class I or III saddles to act as a stop for the purpose of establishing the vertical dimension; and there are Class II saddles which must be used for the purpose of recording centric and other relations.

For bounded saddles, therefore, where movement of the saddles cannot take place, softened wax is added, the denture inserted, and the patient asked to close. If a free-end saddle is present, a 'V' notch is made in the rim and a quick-setting plaster or zinc oxide impression paste added to this surface prior to the patient closing. A fluid material must be used to prevent the overcompression of the tissues under the saddle.

Plastic partial dentures

Where plastic partial dentures are being con-structed, it is essential to record the centric jaw relationship using occlusal rims on temporary bases as outlined in Chapter 2. The technique of recording occlusion is exactly the same as for a metal denture. The occlusal rims can then be used in exactly the same way for mounting the master casts (Figure 13.2 and Chapter 6).

Functional occlusal pathways

In some cases where one jaw has a complete complement of natural teeth, which have an

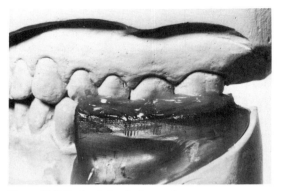

Figure 13.2 Occlusal rims being used to mount master casts

irregular form, it is possible to generate a functional occlusal form in the opposing occlusal rim rather than to attempt to set up the occlusion on the articulator. In order to do this it is essential to have the final impression of the free-end saddles in a functional form, as previously described. The occlusal rim is produced at a slightly higher level than required, with a hard wax, and the patient then grinds on the wax rim until a balanced occlusal form is produced (Figure 13.3).

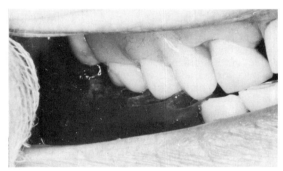

Figure 13.3 A hard wax rim used to generate functional occlusal pathways

The occlusal form which has been generated may be reproduced by the technician in acrylic resin. If an opposing surface is cast to the wax this may be used to articulate stock teeth which have been ground to fit into the opposing cast. The grinding of the acrylic or porcelain teeth to fit the occlusal template is time-consuming, as is the whole technique, and it is not one which is widely used.

Selection of anterior teeth

In difficult cases it is advisable to select the actual teeth to be used at the chairside and decide if any staining is to be carried out. In routine cases, however, a shade is taken by matching the natural teeth to a shade guide. It may be necessary to use shade guides of various manufacturers before one is found to fit the patient's needs. The shade is particularly important in anterior teeth, but in most cases the mould can be selected by the laboratory technician from the standing teeth on the cast.

If all the six natural anterior teeth have been lost the artificial ones are selected on the same basis as for complete dentures.

Selection of posterior teeth

The posterior teeth are usually selected by the technician according to the length of the saddles and the occlusion. In some cases the occlusion may have already been decided at the design stage and a provisional 'set-up' made. These teeth would then be available to complete the setting up of the denture.

If the occlusal surfaces of the upper teeth have been markedly changed since the study casts were taken, a further facebow recording will be required together with any lateral or protrusive records to adjust the articulator. In most cases these are not necessary since the facebow recording can be obtained from the study casts and the adjustment of the articulator settings will be the same as for the study casts.

An occlusal transfer index

If a new facebow recording has not been taken, the study casts are used to prepare an occlusal transfer index, or a facebow recording is taken from the articulator. To prepare an occlusal transfer index, the lower study cast is removed and the upper cast coated with a plaster separating material. A cylinder of wax is shaped around the lower mounting plate and filled with plaster to a level 3 mm above the occlusal plane (Figure 13.4). The articulator is then closed to allow the teeth on the upper cast to make shallow indentations in the soft plaster which, when set, is used to remount the master cast in exactly the same position as the study cast. If only a few teeth are present then an occlusal rim will be necessary and the one used to mount the study cast can be used again for this purpose, provided that the fit on the master cast is satisfactory.

Mounting master casts on the articulator

If an occlusal transfer index is not available the upper cast is mounted by means of a facebow as described previously for study casts. The lower cast

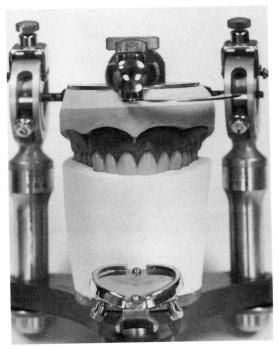

Figure 13.4 Occlusal transference index fixed to the lower arm of the articulator

is then mounted in planned centric occlusion. The articulator is adjusted to give the lateral movements by reference to the wear facets on the teeth. If insufficient teeth or facets are available, lateral and protrusive records must be used to set the articulator variables or if this has been carried out with study casts the same settings may be used.

Tooth arrangement

This is often difficult in partial dentures owing to the drifting and unevenness of the occlusion and it requires some experience in selecting the type and number of teeth to be placed on a saddle. Since grinding of the teeth is often necessary, acrylic resin teeth are to be preferred.

Articulation

Balanced articulation envisages all the teeth in contact in all closed jaw relations, thus stabilizing the dentures. Perfect balance is unlikely in partial dentures, but since the maximum masticatory load is usually on the working side, as wide a contact as possible should be provided in the working-side occlusion.

Buccolingual positioning

The artificial teeth are subject to pressures, in the same way as the natural teeth, from the tongue on the one side and the buccinator and orbicularis oris on the other. If the soft tissues have moulded the natural teeth into positions of stability, it is essential to position the artificial teeth in a similar manner. In partial dentures this is not usually a difficult procedure and failures due to faulty positioning are rare. If the remaining natural teeth and the jaw relations suggest that the lost teeth were in cross-bite, then the artificial teeth should copy this relationship.

Anteroposterior relationship

It is not essential to position all the artificial teeth on the denture as a matter of routine. Only sufficient are necessary to provide an adequate occlusion. When positioning teeth adjacent to the minor connectors, the contact should be ground to obtain a good adaptation.

Aesthetic considerations

Personalization of teeth by the addition of fillings is often necessary and can easily be carried out with acrylic resin teeth. With the wide range of artificial teeth at present on sale, it is seldom that a suitable tooth cannot be found and modified, but failing this teeth can be individually made.

If fillings are required, a hole is drilled from the lingual side of the tooth without breaking through the surface labially and interproximally and the necessary self-curing resin is added to fill the cavity. When set it is polished down and a most satisfactory result occurs. Porcelain teeth may be modified and stained in a similar manner but the technique is more time-consuming. The porcelain tooth is ground slightly to remove the glaze, and stain to represent the filling is painted on to the surface which, when dry, is coated with a low-fusing clear porcelain glaze and then fired at the necessary temperature. Inlays can also be made and cemented into either acrylic or porcelain teeth.

Where resorption of the alveolus has been very minimal, teeth may be ground and fitted directly on to the gum without a flange. These gum-fitted teeth may be aesthetic, but the effect depends on the line of the gingival margins, and if it is obvious that the gingival papillae are missing, the effect will be poor.

Wax contouring

Since retention is not dependent on the peripheral seal of a partial denture, the periphery can be determined in a more arbitrary manner than in complete dentures. In waxing up the saddle it is as well to extend to the borders of the cast and to cut back, where necessary, any over-extension in the clinic. The contours of the wax would be as simple as possible in the posterior region, with no elaborate gingival contouring. In the anterior region, however, the gingival contour should be as exact as possible. Ideally, the anterior saddles should be shaped to blend with the soft tissues (Figure 13.5).

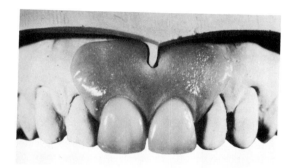

Figure 13.5 The anterior wax flange of a denture correctly contoured to restore the soft tissues

The eye is always quick to observe discontinuities of line and height of tissues and any break in the natural level of the gingival margins makes the teeth look artificial. These areas should not be undercut, relative to the insertion path of the denture, since they should have been eliminated by surveying the cast in a tilted position (see p. 140). The metal framework is prepared with finishing lines so that the acrylic resin forms a butt joint with the saddle and it is preferable, therefore, to wax up these with a slight excess in order to allow for trimming down of the acrylic when it is processed. Care must be taken in waxing around the teeth to ensure that small grooves which would retain stains, etc. around the necks of the teeth are eliminated but the technique is essentially the same as for complete dentures.

When complete, the denture is removed from the cast and cleaned and it may then be reseated on the cast and sent for final trial.

The final trial of the denture

In the clinic the dentures should be washed with soap and water prior to insertion. All the features relating to the denture are checked to ensure that when processed they will be satisfactory. In metal partial dentures the framework has already been assessed and corrected impressions recorded. The dentures should be stable and not rock on pressure. They should fit accurately and the occlusion of the natural and artificial teeth should be such as to give even contact of all the occluding teeth in centric occlusion. The patient should be asked to approve the aesthetics before the dentures are returned to the laboratory.

Where plastic partial dentures are being constructed, the same criteria apply in that the temporary base and the artificial teeth are placed in the patient's mouth and the occlusion and aesthetics checked in exactly the same way as for a metal denture.

14

Processing of complete and partial dentures

When a satisfactory try-in has been completed and the dentures returned to the laboratory, the wax part must be converted into acrylic resin. With partial dentures the occlusion is checked on the articulator but with complete dentures, if an adjustable articulator has been used set to average values, it will be necessary to loosen the condylar controls and place the lateral and protrusive records in between the trial dentures and adjust the condylar settings for the individual records in the same manner as that described in Chapter 7, page 55. With complete dentures the centre bearing point is removed together with the records and with the articulator set for individual values the occlusion of the dentures can now be corrected and finalized.

When finalized the wax is smoothed and, as with metal partial dentures, the peripheral wax edges are sealed down to the cast with molten wax to prevent the plaster, used to invest the denture, from creeping under the edges and spoiling the cast surface.

With acrylic resin partial dentures the master cast is preferably duplicated whilst the wax blocking out undercuts is present to create a working cast upon which the trial denture is transferred. The trial dentures sealed down to the cast are now ready for investing.

Investing or flasking

A flask is a metal sectional box used for holding the plaster mould of the waxed-up denture into which the acrylic resin is packed. Flasking is the procedure of investing the waxed-up denture in a flask to produce a sectional mould. The process allows pressure to be developed in the acrylic resin as it is confined within the mould. The flask is usually in two sections, one part being deeper than the other,

and in some cases the top or bottom of each section can be removed (Figure 14.1). The selection of a good flask is important and the flask should be made of a good quality alloy so that distortion and bending are prevented. They should never be subjected to

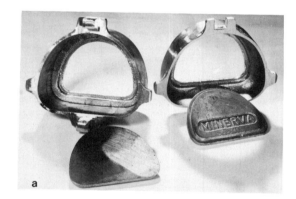

a

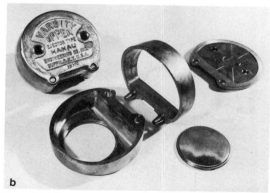

b

Figure 14.1 Two types of flask. Note that the inserts for (a) fit inside the flask. In (b) one part fits on the outside

hammering with an iron hammer. Poor flasks, which allow movement between the sections and do not fit together correctly, lead to changes in the occlusion of the finished dentures.

The procedure employed for flasking complete and partial dentures is slightly different and each is described separately.

Complete dentures – flasking procedure

(1) Remove the wax dentures on their casts from the articulator split-cast mounting plaster. If heat-cured bases have been employed, the plaster casts poured to the bases are treated in exactly the same way as temporary bases.

(2) Paint sodium alginate separating solution onto the base and sides of the cast and lubricate the inside of the flask with Vaseline. This will make deflasking procedures easier.

(3) Fill two-thirds of the shallow part of the flask with a mix of plaster. Settle the upper cast with the waxed-up denture into this plaster. Excess plaster will extrude up and over the flask rims. Centre the denture in the plaster and keep the anterior section slightly higher than the posterior section. Trim off the excess plaster with a plaster knife, and smooth the plaster with water while it is still soft. Make sure that no undercuts exist and that there is a smooth transition of plaster between the rim of the flask and the land area of the cast (Figure 14.2). The upper and lower are dealt with in the same way, but with the lower make certain there is sufficient plaster to support the retromolar pad areas of the cast and allow the plaster to extend over the tongue area of the cast so that all undercuts are eliminated.

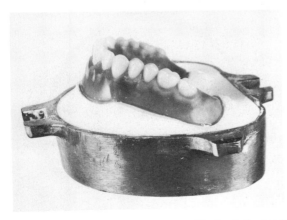

Figure 14.2 The upper denture mounted in the shallow part of the flask

(4) After the plaster in the shallow part of the flask is set, paint a separating medium over all the exposed plaster and stone surfaces. This is to ensure that the second part of the mould will not adhere.

(5) Prepare a mix of equal parts of plaster and stone with water and paint part of it over the teeth and waxed-up denture, using a small amount of vibration to avoid entrapping air bubbles. The rest of the mix is placed into the deep part of the flask and the shallow part inverted onto the deep part and the two halves pressed together to ensure the flasks are in good contact. This method requires some experience in judging the right consistency of the mix to manage the inversion and closing of the flask. Alternatively, a two-stage topping procedure may be used. With this technique, a thin coating (approx. 6 mm) of stone is applied to the teeth and waxwork and allowed to set. The deeper half of the flask is filled with plaster, and the shallow half of the flask with the already set stone capping is inverted onto the deep section and the flask closed.

With some flasks, within which the top section can be removed, the deep part of the flask is placed *in situ* over the shallow part and a mix of plaster/stone is poured directly onto the teeth and wax into the flask until it is full, and then closed off with a flask lid.

(6) Allow the top half of the mould to set completely.

Partial dentures – flasking procedure

When flasking partial dentures, it is preferable to arrange for all the acrylic resin to be placed into one part of the flask, as it is with complete dentures. The working cast and the denture base are embedded in the shallow section of the flask with the lower part of the wax periphery level with the top edges of the flask (Figure 14.3). When the deep part of the flask is fitted over the top and filled with an equal mix of plaster and stone, the saddle will be entirely in this part. When separated and the wax removed, the teeth will be retained in the deep section of the flask and all the acrylic resin material can then be packed into this part. This is better than embedding half the denture in each part of the flask, since the junction of the two pieces of acrylic resin would join on the side of the denture and a line may be seen when it is completed. The procedure to be adopted for flasking partials is obviously similar to that used in complete dentures. However, the subtle differences should be noted.

The flask should be big enough to allow at least 13 mm of space around the cast and the denture in all places. The working cast may be trimmed down

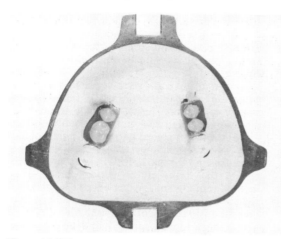

Figure 14.3 The partial denture flasked

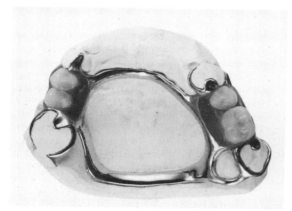

Figure 14.4 A master cast being reduced on a model trimmer and the stone teeth reduced in height

on a model grinder and the stone teeth reduced in height (Figure 14.4). The cast is located with the periphery of the cast level with the metal flange. All other parts of the cast are covered with plaster.

Gum-fitted teeth

Gum-fitted teeth are retained on the denture base by hooding with plaster (Figure 14.5) and therefore not withdrawn into the opposite half of the flask when the wax is removed.

Complete and partial dentures – removal of the wax pattern

In order to separate the wax from the teeth and allow the two sections of the flask to be opened, the flask is immersed in water at a temperature of 100°C

for 5 minutes. During this time the wax will become soft and the two halves of the flask can be gently separated. The softened wax should be lifted out in one piece, if possible, and all the teeth, unless they have been hooded, will be left in the upper section of the flask. On no account should the heating process result in the wax becoming molten as this soaks into the plaster, making the following stages exceedingly difficult. Residual wax should be flushed out with boiling water, to which has been added a detergent solution (2% Teepol). Wax prevents penetration of the separating material onto the plaster and also prevents bonding of the teeth to the resin.

Finally, the flask is flushed with clean hot water and then allowed to drain. Any teeth that have become loose must be carefully replaced into the mould. If a relief is necessary, the soft metal (0.25 mm) should be glued into place over the prescribed area. Trim the edges of the plaster at the periphery to remove any small, thin edges which may break away when packing and become incorporated in the acrylic resin.

Separation

When the mould is dry, alginate separating material is painted onto the surface of the plaster and stone in both sections of the flask. Failure to apply separating material correctly allows the acrylic resin to penetrate the top layer of plaster or stone and, when deflasked, the denture will be covered in a plaster or stone surface. Removal of this is exceedingly difficult and the contours of denture are spoilt. Tin foil is the best separating material, but this is somewhat difficult and time-consuming to

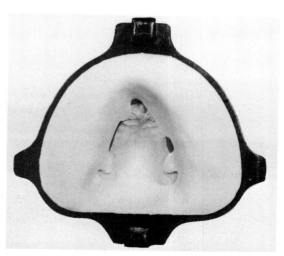

Figure 14.5 Gum-fitted teeth hooded with plaster in the deep part of the flask

apply and, in practice, an alginate material is satisfactory for most purposes.

If tin foil is to be used, it is preferable to apply it to the waxed-up surface of the dentures prior to flasking and, when the wax is removed, it is already held in the top part of the flask. At this stage, therefore, only the cast surface has to be tin-foiled. When using clear acrylics, tin foil will ensure a superior result.

[If the denture requires a post-dam, a check is made that this has been prepared in the cast.]

Preparation of the acrylic resin

It is essential to ensure complete cleanliness in packing a denture and preferably this should be carried out in a room set aside for the purposes of packing and polymerizing of the acrylic resin. Personal cleanliness is also important, and the same precautions in relation to monomer as that decribed in Chapter 3 and in Appendix VII must be followed.

The powder or polymer is mixed with the liquid monomer in a ratio between 3:1 and 3.5:1 by volume. This is essential to allow a thorough wetting and solution of the polymer granules. Some variations will occur depending on the type of powder and the manufacturers' recommendations. Usually, for a complete denture 32 ml of powder and 10 ml of monomer are used. The liquid is added to a clean porcelain jar or a polythene pot and the polymer added until all the liquid is taken up. Since the dye is added to the surface of the granules, care must be taken to see that streaks of colour do not develop in the resin as the granules dissolve in the monomer. The mixture is stirred, covered with a lid,

and allowed to stand until it has passed from a wet sand stage, through a stringy, sticky stage and on into a dough or putty-like stage. The time taken to reach this stage will depend, in the main, upon: (1) the shape and size of the granule, (2) the molecular weight of the polymer, (3) the temperature, and (4) the powder:liquid ratio. The ideal material will reach the dough stage rapidly, but will stay in the dough stage for a long time to enable packing to take place without undue pressure. In hot weather, it can be controlled by refrigeration and in cold weather, by warming the mixing pot.

Packing

When the dough has reached a non-sticky state, it is rolled into a ball, packed into the deep section of the flask, and pressed out to overfill the mould. The flask containing the cast is inverted over the deep part and closed together with hand pressure and then placed in a hydraulic press and closed very slowly. The pressure applied must not exceed 4×10^5 Pa. It is essential to close the flask slowly and have the dough in the correct state as excess pressure may drive the teeth into the plaster or crack the cast. Most acrylic resins do not require trial closures if the flow properties of the dough are satisfactory. However, in extra thick cases, if the operator prefers a trial closure, it may be used. When undertaking trial closures, the dough is packed into the deep section of the flask and pressed out to overfill the mould. The mixing jar is kept covered to prevent evaporation of the monomer. A sheet of cellophane or polythene is placed over the flask which is closed under pressure. The flasks are

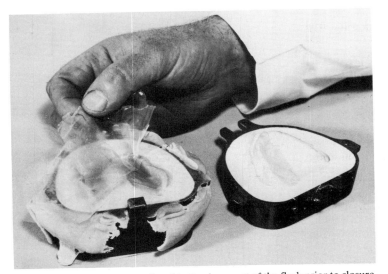

Figure 14.6 The acrylic resin placed in the deep part of the flask prior to closure

then removed from the hydraulic press and opened carefully; the cellophane or polythene film is removed, and excess acrylic is trimmed off with a sharp carver (Figure 14.6). Add a small amount of fresh, clean dough to the mould and repeat the trial closure again. Re-open the flask the second time and remove the excess material. Cover the flask with a film of cellophane to prevent evaporation of the monomer from the acrylic resin and paint the cast with a separating solution. When dry, remove the covering cellophane from the packed part of the flask and close together. When partial dentures are being packed, it is not always possible to carry out this procedure and each case must be treated individually. For instance, when a metal saddle is present, it is necessary to pack some acrylic around the frame of the saddle in addition to that in the deep part of the flask (Figure 14.7). Cellophane or

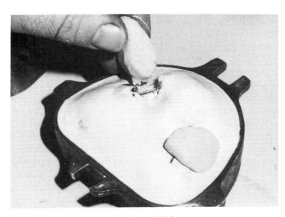

Figure 14.7 Packing a metal partial denture

polythene film is placed over each half when trial packing. This is necessary or the acrylic would engage the retention bars and pull out of the deep part of the flask when opened after the first trial packing.

Partial dentures with some teeth held in the lower part, whilst the others are in the upper part of the flask, are packed in the same manner, except that the separating solution is applied to each section to be packed at the beginning of the process. The dough is mixed and packed into each section of the flask, and in some cases where a flange is present in the region of the hooded teeth, it is preferable to remove the teeth from the flask and pack the acrylic through into the flange area and then reposition the teeth before packing the remainder. It is seldom necessary to do this and, where possible, this difficult process should be avoided. Gum fitting the teeth simplifies the packing procedure if they are hooded.

When the flask is packed, a separating film of cellophane or polythene is placed between the two sections of the flask and a trial closure made. The precedure is then similar to that previously described. Once flasks are finally closed and metal-to-metal contact has been achieved, they must be kept in a closed position whilst the acrylic resin is polymerized. They must be removed from the press and placed in a spring clamp, which is tightened and keeps the flask under spring pressure during the polymerizing stage (Figure 14.8).

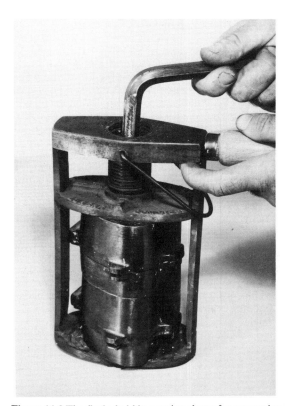

Figure 14.8 The flasks held in a spring clamp for processing

Strengtheners

Acrylic resin has a relatively poor flexural fatigue and impact strengths and, in many cases, fractures occur with serious results. In order to avoid this, some strengthening of the material with glass fibre, metal gauze or nylon has been advocated. The danger is greater because acrylic resin is radiolucent and therefore if inhaled or swallowed it is not possible to identify on the X-ray film. Attempts have been made to make it radio-opaque with various barium compounds, but without a great deal of success. The insertion of metal mesh is not very satisfactory as it is said to weaken the material, but does hold the pieces together if fracture occurs. Nylon gauze, likewise, is not wetted by the acrylic resin and is therefore unsatisfactory. With both these materials it is probable that the acrylic resin shrinks away from the 'strengthening' material and therefore one has an acrylic material with a network of holes which naturally weakens the structure.

Fibreglass mesh or wool or carbon fibre can be used, but it is difficult to pack enough material into the finished product to increase its strength greatly. If gauze is used, several layers are needed and are best laid between sheets of resin before packing in the flask. This is, however, a difficult process to produce a satisfactory result and in many cases the gauze comes to the surface of the denture and polishing is rendered difficult. If increased strength is necessary, the denture should be made in metal or constructed in one of the higher impact resistant rubber added acrylic resins which give an impact strength approximately three times that of conventional denture acrylics.

In order to prevent the swallowing or inhaling of the denture, the plate should be large enough to prevent it from going into the pharynx.

Staining of dentures

In order to improve the appearance of dentures, it is possible to shade the acrylic resin to appear similar to the natural gingival tissues. It will be observed, when examining a patient, that the eminences over the roots of the teeth are somewhat lighter in colour than the rest of the tissues, whilst the interdental papillae are slightly darker. Also, there are often pigmented areas and blood vessels to be seen, all of which can be reproduced in the acrylic resin denture. The acrylics used for this purpose are of a fine particle size and the colouring pigment is distributed throughout the granules. Several stains and shades of pink are available. It is usual to have a shade guide available in the clinic and to make a sketch indicating where the various shades are needed.

A separating solution must be carefully applied to the area concerned. The fine nozzles on the bottles are used to position the powder carefully on the mould surface which will be the labial surface of the denture (Figure 14.9). Once the powder has been placed in position, monomer is added to the powder with a fine pipette to dampen the material. Care must be taken not to add too much or the material will flow out of the correct position. This process is repeated on all the areas which need staining and small red nylon or PVC threads can be incorporated to give the appearance of blood vessels. The surface of the plaster mould is covered with a thin film of

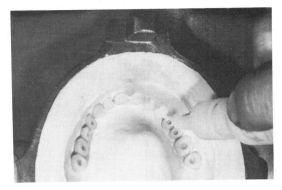

Figure 14.9 Kayon powders being applied to the stone cast

stains and then the normal acrylic is packed into place. The resulting denture has a very natural appearance.

If staining is not carried out as part of the processing of the denture, stains are available for painting on the denture (Minute Stains) after processing.

Soft lining materials

Some patients experience pain from dentures if they load the underlying mucosa on sharp bony ridges. This is usually a greater problem in the mandible than the maxilla owing to the smaller area of bone supporting the denture, and soft plastics have been used in an attempt to overcome this problem.

These materials are either based on the higher esters of methacrylic acid, together with plasticizers, or are silicone elastomers. Both are supplied in the autopolymerizing form, or may be heat cured in a manner similar to the denture base. The esters bond well, but have a poor clinical life, whilst the autopolymerizing silicones are difficult to bond to the methyl methacrylate resins. The heat cure type are usually satisfactory and have a long clinical life.

After the normal boiling out procedure, when a denture is being made, a layer of wax is placed over the cast to the same thickness that is required for the soft plastics. The denture is then packed with normal acrylic in the usual way and, after the first trial closure, the spacing material is removed and the soft lining is packed into the mould on top of the normal material. Cellophane or polythene is then applied and a second trial closure made. The procedure is then as for a normal denture.

In packing the viscous heat cured silicone materials, it is often wise to allow the packed denture and spacing material to stand in the press for several hours in order to allow the resin to become hard before packing the lining material.

Failure to do so prevents sufficient pressure being developed when packing the lining and porosity may result.

Polymerization/processing/curing

These terms are synonymous. There are a variety of curing cycles that may be employed, most manufacturers recommend two or three different curing cycles, and either wet or dry heat may be used.

The dimensional changes associated with converting the monomer to polymer using a heating cycle result in the final denture being slightly smaller than the cast. This tendency can be minimized by using the lowest possible curing temperature. The initiation of the conversion of the monomer to polymer by the benzoyl peroxide will take place at about 70°C and any heating above this temperature will have an adverse effect on the dimensional accuracy of the denture base since thermal contraction must occur on cooling to room temperature. High levels of residual monomer can have a deleterious effect on denture base polymers but can be reduced to a minimum by a terminal boil of at least 1 hour.

This terminal boil, however, must not be carried out until the bulk of the monomer is converted or porosity may result. Thus, it is necessary that some compromise is required to obtain good dimensional accuracy, minimal levels of monomer and porous free dentures. A curing cycle of 7 hours at 70°C, plus 1 hour at 100°C is considered to be the best practical curing cycle. It provides porosity-free dentures, gives residual monomer levels of less than 1.0% and the additional shrinkage as a consequence of the terminal boil is too small (less than 0.2%) to have any clinical relevance. It should, however, be noticed that when using most commercially available water baths that it takes more than 1 hour for the temperature to rise from 70°C to 100°C, depending upon the volume of water and the number of flasks being processed. Thus, when using water baths the timing clocks should be set at 7 hours at 70°C (delayed) and 3 hours at 100°C. This curing cycle is satisfactory for all heat curing polymers and soft lining materials.

Deflasking

The flasks, when removed from the processing tank, are allowed to bench cool to room temperature. The flasks are then removed from the spring clamp. The removal of the polymerized denture from the plaster mould can be difficult owing to the hardness of the plaster and care must be taken to avoid damage to the denture. The first stage is to remove the investing plaster in one block from the flask and this may be brought about by gently tapping the base in

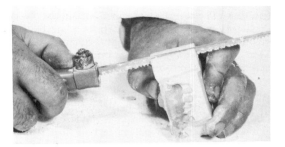

Figure 14.10 Removing the outer layer of gypsum with a keyhole saw

the bottom of each section of the flask with a rubber mallet. A 'ball' of plaster is then left with the denture inside. The investing plaster surrounding the cast is separated using a keyhole saw (Figure 14.10) and a knife to remove the plaster from the denture (Figure 14.11). This stage is generally easily achieved if the cast has been coated with sodium alginate as suggested previously. The remaining plaster mould is then carefully sectioned by inserting a knife blade between them and prising them from the denture. It is important to remember in complete denture construction, where the split cast technique has been used, that the denture should be left on the cast at this stage.

Elimination of processing errors

When acrylic resin is packed in the flask and processed, dimensional changes take place which cause errors in the occlusion of the denture. The following are some of the possible causes of laboratory processing errors:

(1) The wax may change dimension during flasking.

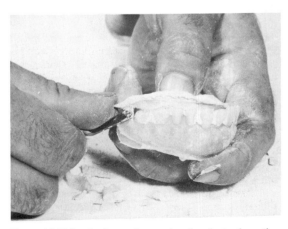

Figure 14.11 Sectioning and removing the plaster from the completed denture

(2) The teeth may be forced into the plaster owing to the packing pressure.

(3) Badly fitting sections of the flask will prevent correction orientation of the teeth to the cast.

(4) Thermal and polymerizing changes take place in the resin.

Whilst these are the major causes of error, there are others which may possibly arise during the processing stage and it is essential to correct these laboratory errors.

The dentures, when processed on split casts, should now be fitted onto the mounting cups of the articulator and any errors in the occlusion can be observed. Movement of the teeth in the flask usually causes the master casts to be held apart. The incisal guidance pin on the articulator will stand away from the incisal guidance table and the artificial teeth must be ground to restore the planned occlusion (Figure 14.12).

Selective grinding of complete dentures

Grinding of the occlusal surfaces of the artificial teeth at selected points is carried out to ensure that the centric occlusion of the teeth coincides with the centric jaw relation and also that the dentures have balanced eccentric contact in all positions. Elimination of the deflective contacts of the teeth with provision of balanced occlusion is one of the most important stages in the fabrication of dentures whether carried out as a laboratory procedure at this stage or as a clinical remount after the dentures have been tried in the patient. It is an exacting process and takes some time to complete correctly, and before beginning to carry it out a thorough understanding of balanced occlusion is necessary. This procedure is mainly to correct minor errors in clinical and/or laboratory procedures. It is not a means of eliminating gross errors where an incorrect centric relation has been recorded.

The procedure is carried out in two stages:

(1) The correction of the centric occlusion at the correct centric relation and vertical dimension.

(2) The development of eccentric balancing contacts.

The correction of centric occlusion

The condylar mechanism is locked on the articulator so that it works as a hinge mechanism. The teeth are tapped lightly together with a piece of thin carbon articulating paper between them. Any black spots produced would indicate premature contacts in this relation. Before grinding it will be necessary to ensure that these points will not be required for eccentric contact (Figure 14.13). The articulator is freed again for this purpose and the position of the teeth with these contacts is observed in the working and balancing side position. If preferred, a second coloured articulating paper can be used to record the eccentric high spots in addition to the centric ones. Three rules must be observed during this stage of grinding: (a) If a cusp is high in both centric and eccentric positions reduce the cusp. (b) If a cusp is high in centric but not in eccentric occlusion deepen the fossa. (c) If a cusp is high in eccentric only, it

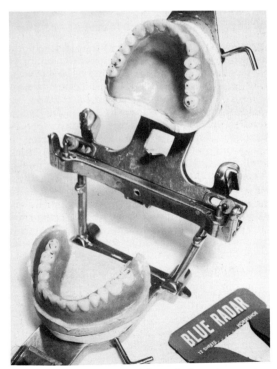

Figure 14.13 Examination of the occlusion necessary to ensure that occlusal contacts at centric relation are not reduced if they are required in eccentric movements

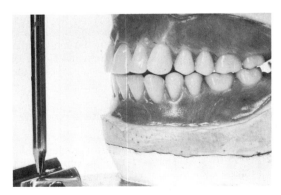

Figure 14.12 Remounted dentures. Note the errors in occlusion leading to the incisal guidance pin being raised

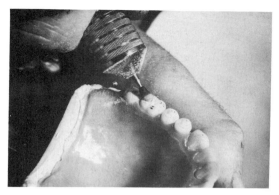

Figure 14.14 Grinding of the occlusal surfaces is carried out with a small carborundum stone

must be left at this stage since only centric contacts are being considered.

The grinding is carried out with a small carborundum stone in a handpiece, doing small sections at a time (Figure 14.14). Identification of the areas to be ground is repeated until eventually the incisal guidance pin fits on to the incisal guidance table. At this stage, the buccal cusps of all the lower teeth and the fossa of all the upper teeth should have black contact spots.

The development of eccentric contacts

It is essential now to follow certain rules in the grinding to avoid destroying the centric occlusion and the following rules must always be borne in mind: (a) Do not reduce the maxillary lingual cusp. (b) Do not reduce the mandibular buccal cusp. (c) Do not deepen the fossa of any tooth. The incisal guidance pin is raised and the eccentric contacts determined by articulating paper. Grinding is carried out in accordance with the above rules, sometimes called BU, LL rule (buccal upper, lingual lower). Careful grinding of only the inclines and the cusp will prevent the aesthetic appearance of the teeth being destroyed. Since two movements are involved, it is necessary to examine the teeth in two positions, namely the working and the balancing positions. For grinding these contacts certain rules are set out as follows:

(1) On the working side, reduce inner inclines of maxillary buccal cusp (Figure 14.15).

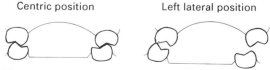

Figure 14.15 The reduction of the inner inclines of the maxillary buccal cusp to produce eccentric contacts

(2) Reduce inner inclines of mandibular lingual cusp (Figure 14.16).

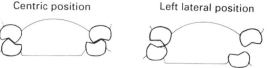

Figure 14.16 The reduction of the mandibular lingual cusp inclines

(3) On the balancing side, reduce inner inclines of the upper palatal or mandibular buccal cusp (Figure 14.17).

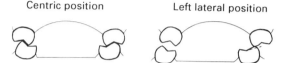

Figure 14.17 The reduction of the inner inclines of the upper palatal or mandibular buccal cusps to achieve balance

If the processing has been carried out carefully, selective grinding should be minimal and little grinding of the incisal teeth, other than the canines, will be required. The changes in the vertical dimension are always such that an increase occurs and the anterior teeth do not come into contact. However, if errors have arisen and selective grinding is carried out, it is essential to preserve the aesthetic appearance of the teeth. If gross changes are needed, it is better to take off the posterior teeth and re-record centric relation and proceed to make a new denture, or reset the posterior teeth.

Protrusion

The rules for grinding in protrusion are as follows: (a) Reduce the distal inclines of the maxillary lingual cusp. (b) Reduce the mesial inclines of the mandibular buccal cusp. (c) Reduce the lingual surfaces of the incisal edges of the upper teeth and the labial surfaces of the edges of the mandibular incisal teeth. (d) Reduce the distolingual slopes of maxillary canines and the mesiobuccal slopes of the mandibular ones.

Selective grinding with a cross-bite in eccentric relation

The normal procedure is adopted for obtaining the correct centric occlusion and the following rules are used for grinding in an eccentric situation which are the reverse of those previously noted: (a) Do not reduce maxillary buccal cusps. (b) Do not reduce mandibular lingual cusps. (c) Do not deepen the fossa of any tooth. The rules for refining the eccentric occlusion are as follows:

(1) On the working side: (a) reduce any inclines of maxillary lingual cusps; (b) reduce inner inclines of mandibular buccal cusps; (c) on the balancing side, reduce the inner inclines of mandibular lingual cusps.
(2) In protrusive relationships: (a) reduce the distal inclines of maxillary buccal cusps; (b) reduce the mesial inclines of the mandibular lingual cusps.

At this stage, the occlusion should be almost perfect and can be finalized by milling in with a carborundum paste. The fine powder can be mixed with glycerine and painted over the teeth and the articulator moved to either side to allow the teeth to rub over one another (Figure 14.18). This is carried out until the movement is smooth and continuous from one eccentric position to another. It should not be carried out to an excessive degree or the cusps will become gradually flattened.

Once the laboratory errors have been eliminated, the dentures are removed from their cast by sectioning the cast using a pad saw and knife.

Selective grinding of partial dentures

Partial dentures must be ground in to provide the occlusion which was anticipated when designing the denture. It will seldom be possible to obtain

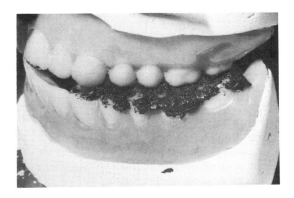

Figure 14.18 The use of fine carborundum to remove irregularities and produce a smooth articulation

balanced articulation in the sense that one obtains this in complete dentures, but the general principles concerned with the grinding of teeth are the same. For this reason, therefore, the process of selective grinding in complete dentures has been described and can be applied to any partial denture situation.

With partial dentures (and complete dentures that have been constructed on working casts and not on the split-cast principle), they can only be selectively ground by remounting after insertion of the dentures with a new centric record.

15

Polishing and finishing acrylic resin

If the separating material has been applied correctly, the surface of the resin should be clean and shiny when deflasked. The initial stage is to remove the excess acrylic resin or flash at the edges of the denture with a stone in a handpiece, followed by sandpaper, to give a smooth surface. Pimples and lumps around the teeth can be removed with a sharp trimmer. The posterior margin of the denture must be trimmed back carefully to the post-dam and the palate thinned if necessary to make the back edge of the denture as inconspicuous to the tongue as possible. Small pimples arise on the surface of the acrylic resin due to the packing pressure breaking down small voids in the stone and forcing in the resin, and these must be smoothed.

With partial dentures, the acrylic resin is trimmed using small stones in a handpiece. Coarse, large stones should not be used as these may inadvertently create deep scratches in the metal denture surface which have to be removed by the use of a series of progressively finer abrasives.

If the processing of the dentures has been carried out carefully, they can almost be polished with pumice once the flash and pimples have been removed. The polishing of dentures consists of making them smooth and glossy without changing their contour. This is achieved by using a variety of sizes and shapes of polishing brushes, wheels and mops with progressively finer degrees of abrasives. It should be noted that variations in abrasive powder are influenced not only by the abrasive used but by pressure and speed also.

The polishing procedure involves holding the denture against a rotating large bristle brush or cloth wheel (Figure 15.1) wet with a slurry of pumice. This rapidly smoothes the large areas of the palate of an upper denture and the periphery in the buccal region. For fine polishing near acrylic resin teeth or

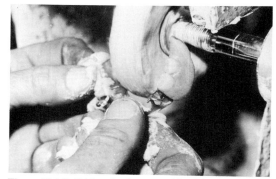

Figure 15.1 Polishing the denture with a felt wheel and a pumice slurry

on labial gum work, a small black bristle brush is substituted for the cloth wheel (Figure 15.2). For this type of polishing, the brush should be reduced to its slowest possible speed to avoid burning the surface. In areas of difficult access, a felt cone may

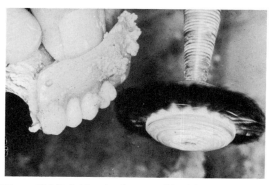

Figure 15.2 Polishing the denture with a black bristle brush

114

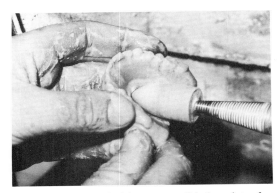

Figure 15.3 The use of a felt cone to polish the palate of a denture

be used to achieve the same result (Figure 15.3) and a small wheel brush in a handpiece can also be useful around the teeth.

The surface of the denture must be continuously moved to avoid excessive abrasion or destruction of the staining and contouring of the gum work and an excess of slurry must always be kept on the denture. Polishing with a cloth wheel with proprietary paste (Tripoli) can then take place in the same way and the final gloss produced on the acrylic resin with a slurry of whiting and water on a cloth mop or soft white wheel brush. These are usually run at high speed and light pressure to achieve the maximum smoothness of surface. Final buffing with a swans-down mop will add a very high lustre.

Acrylic teeth are often polished in error in this process and the beginner is advised to proceed carefully and slowly to avoid the aesthetic appearance being destroyed.

Once the polishing stage is completed, the dentures should be washed in soap and warm water and then stored in an antiseptic solution in a sealed polythene bag until supplied to the patient.

16

Insertion, recall and maintenance of dentures

The denture, after completion, should be returned to the clinic/surgery in a disinfectant and this should be washed off in the sight of the patient.

Insertion of complete dentures

The dentures should be inspected for nodules on the fitting surface. These should be removed together with any rough areas which may cause the patient discomfort. On insertion of the denture every aspect should be considered and re-evaluated. First, the retention should be considered though, at this stage, until the saliva has thoroughly wetted the denture the retention may not be as good as it will be after a few days. Unilateral stability can also be evaluated by pressing on the artificial teeth to ensure that the denture does not become displaced. Assuming that all is satisfactory, the remaining assessment to be made is that centric occlusion and the centric jaw relationship coincide. It is unlikely, at this stage, that this will be perfect as most errors arise due to the clinical procedures rather than the laboratory processing.

In order to achieve a good centric jaw relationship which coincides with the centric occlusion of the dentures and also to achieve balanced articulation and bilateral lateral stability, it is often necessary, at this stage, to re-record the centric jaw relationship and return the dentures to the laboratory for selective grinding to be carried out whilst the patient waits. The recording of centric jaw relationship should be carried out in exactly the same way as when it was first recorded using occlusal rims (Chapter 5). Ideally, a centre bearing point and a soft material, such as plaster of Paris, should be used, but for the majority of practitioners this is impractical and a simpler technique of using softened modelling wax on the lower posterior teeth is an acceptable compromise. The wax must be softened evenly throughout and both sides should be of equal thickness. The lower jaw is guided into the most retruded position and closed to a position just before initial contact of the teeth. The wax is chilled with cold air or water and the lower denture removed. If penetration of the wax has taken place the recording must be retaken, but if it is correct the denture can be chilled again in cold water and re-inserted and the centric jaw relationship confirmed. When the dentures are returned following selective grinding (see pages 111–113), they may be coated on the fitting surface with a pressure indicating paste and placed in the mouth and the patient asked to occlude the teeth and apply gentle pressure. When the dentures are removed any excessive pressure areas will be clearly observed as the denture will be completely clear of paste (Figure 16.1). This can then be gently ground with a small

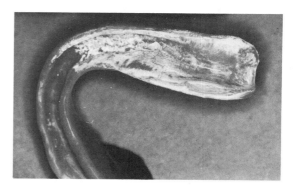

Figure 16.1 The use of a pressure indicating paste in a complete denture to ascertain pressure points under a denture

round carborundum stone and polished. If necessary, this process can be repeated.

Aesthetics must also be evaluated again and the patient presented with a mirror to have a look at the finished product. During this procedure the patient will be able to speak with dentures and evaluation of speech patterns and also the vertical dimension can be made. It may take some time for the patient's muscular activity to become adjusted to the new appliance and the speech will improve after a few days. The patient is given instructions for the maintenance and care of the dentures.

Insertion of partial dentures

The dentures should be washed in the sight of the patient and inserted to ensure that they fit correctly and are retentive and do not move when pressure is applied to the saddles. The occlusion is examined carefully in centric and eccentric positions, but unlike complete dentures, if the dentures are very nearly correct, the teeth may be adjusted by grinding at the chairside. The high points on the teeth are marked with red or blue foils in centric and eccentric positions using a different colour for each procedure and then the high points may be ground using very small carborundum points. On completion, the teeth are polished using a polishing brush and pumice.

The aesthetics of the denture are also examined and the patient's approval obtained. The saddles are coated with pressure indicating paste and any parts showing excessive pressure are lightly ground and polished in exactly the same way as for complete dentures.

If, however, there is considerable discrepancy in the occlusion it is necessary to remount the dentures in the laboratory where grinding can take place or to remove some posterior teeth and replace them by new teeth, attaching them to the base with autopolymerizing resin. A new facebow record will be required with the dentures in place together with the record of centric jaw relationship in exactly the same way as that for study casts (see page 9). If master casts are available, then the dentures can be replaced on the cast and these can be re-articulated. If, however, master casts are not available or are damaged, the procedure for remounting is as follows.

The dentures are inserted and alginate impressions are taken of the maxilla and the mandible with the partial dentures in place. When the impressions are removed they will contain the dentures and the technician will dry the impressions with a blast of air and pour in either hard dye stone or molten Melottes metal to fill the impressions of the natural teeth. Melottes metal is a eutectic alloy which has a

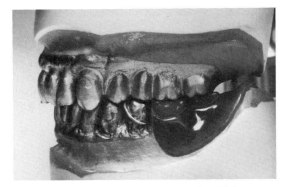

Figure 16.2 The partial denture mounted on Melottes metal cast

low melting point but is reasonably hard and will not chip like ordinary stone used for making casts (Figure 16.2). While still soft retaining wires are added to the metal and the rest of the cast poured in stone. These casts and the dentures can then be mounted on the articulator with the interocclusal and facebow records in the usual way.

Selective grinding of partial dentures

Partial dentures must be ground to provide an occlusion which was anticipated when designing the denture. It will seldom be possible to obtain balanced articulation in the sense that one obtains this in complete dentures, but the general principles concerned with the grinding of the teeth are the same. The movement pattern of the jaws will however be controlled by the guidance of the existing natural teeth and the partial denture must conform to this.

Maintenance and aftercare of dentures

Once the dentures have been inserted and the patient made comfortable a further appointment is made and the patient instructed to return in a few days' time.

It is seldom advisable to give patients detailed instructions at this time as they seldom are able to remember the details. For this reason, it is always preferable to remind the patient with a set of written instructions, and these are shown in Appendix VI.

Patients should be advised to wear the dentures as much as possible before the next appointment but, if soreness develops, to remove the dentures and re-insert them at least 24 hours before the appointment so that sore areas can be identified. During this adjustment appointment the patient should be advised that where complete dentures are concerned they should return for an evaluation at least every year whilst with partial dentures a much more detailed observation must be maintained.

It can be adequately demonstrated in clinical trials that have taken place that the patient should return at 3-monthly intervals for scaling and polishing and that there should be an evaluation each time as to whether periodontal disease or caries is developing. The partial denture can be evaluated at the same time. In certain circumstances where the patient's oral hygiene is excellent and a stable condition exists, longer periods of time may be allowed between visits but this should be essentially a decision made by the dentist with his knowledge of that particular patient.

17

Miscellaneous techniques

The relevance of previous dentures

Most elderly patients who require new dentures will have already been wearing dentures for long periods of time. In adapting to the new dentures the patient may well experience difficulties especially if the polished surface is quite unlike the shape of the old denture and if the occlusal plane level is very much different. During the period since the old dentures were fitted the patient has formed a subtle appreciation of the position of the teeth, the shape of the polished surfaces, and the nature and timing of tooth contact. Having once acquired, with their old dentures, the muscular skill to adapt to denture wearing, the adaptation to new patterns of muscular activity is very difficult.

Thus, as more elderly patients are likely to require replacement dentures, it is important for the technician to have available a technique for copying the shape of dentures. Far too often, inadequate data are given to the technician to copy the old dentures. Impressions of the dentures are often sent to the laboratory to give the technician information concerning the width and shape of the arches and the contours of the polished surfaces, but these fail to indicate the spatial relationship between the teeth and the underlying edentulous ridges.

Three techniques for producing replicas of the patient's old dentures, which may be used as a guide when providing new dentures, are described. The choice of technique will depend upon clinical and laboratory time and facilities available, and the precision of the copy dentures required as well as personal preference.

Copy dentures (Figure 17.1)

Technique 1

Any corrections to the denture periphery may be made with greenstick compound and then a two-part silicone putty mould is prepared. The fitting surface is pressed on to a mass of silicone held in a box or impression tray or other container of suitable shape. When the first half of the mould is set (Figure 17.2) locating notches are carved and Vaseline is applied as a separator and the second half of the mould, an impression of the non-fitting surface, is taken. This process is similar to that in the construction of complete dentures in the flasking stage. Optosil kneadable silicone impression material is ideal for making the mould.

The two halves of the mould are separated and the denture removed and cleaned and returned to the patient. Molten wax is then poured into the tooth portion of the mould (Figure 17.3) and the rest of the mould filled with autopolymerizing resin pressed in at the soft dough stage (Figure 17.4). The two halves of the mould are pressed together and then opened so that the surplus resin may be removed. The mould halves are again closed and held firmly together and placed in a pressure vessel.

Once the replica dentures are cured the flash is trimmed off and also any undercuts from the denture which would prevent removal from the master cast when the impressions have been taken. A failing of this technique is that the acrylic resin base may become thicker than the original base due to distortion of the mould under pressure (Figure 17.5). This will cause the upper anterior teeth to be lower and more labially placed, thus changing the appearance of the denture and also the occlusion. To avoid this a shellac base can be laid as for any denture base on the cast and then the two parts of the mould placed together without pressure, and molten wax poured in through sprue holes to form the teeth and attach them to the base (Figure 17.6).

In recording the centric jaw relationships wax may be added to the occlusal surfaces if adjustments are required. Also, if for aesthetic or functional reasons a change in lip support is required, then again, wax may be added or removed to indicate the amount of

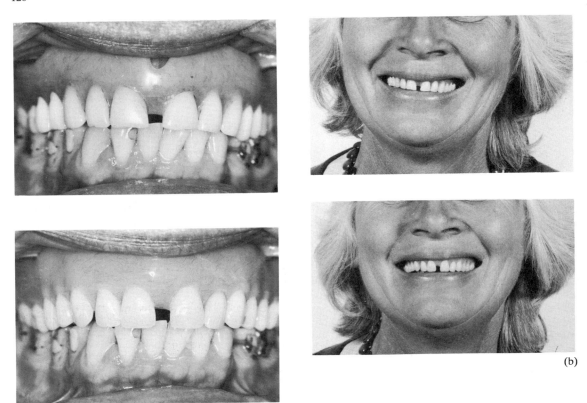

(a)

(b)

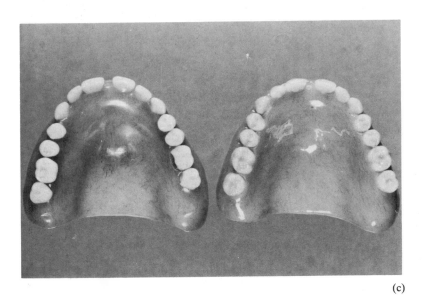

(c)

Figure 17.1 A maxillary copy denture. (a) Upper, before;
lower, after. (b) Upper, before; lower, after. (c) Left, old;
right, new

change required. In Figure 17.7 the replica dentures have been used to take the impressions and record the centric jaw relationship.

After the casts have been poured the replicas are mounted onto the articulator in the usual way.

The setting-up consists of cutting out the wax teeth on the trial base and setting up the new

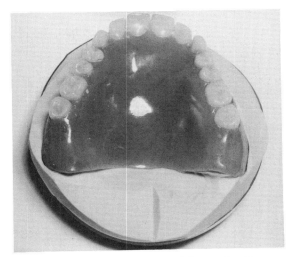

Figure 17.2 A silicone elastomer model created on the fitting surface in one half of the mould

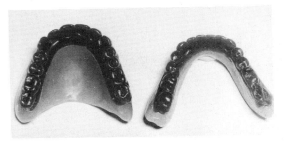

Figure 17.5 Autopolymerizing base and wax teeth forming the denture

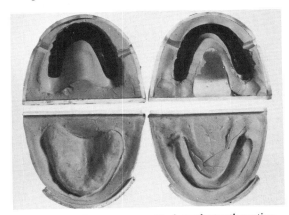

Figure 17.3 Molten wax poured to form the tooth portion of the trial denture

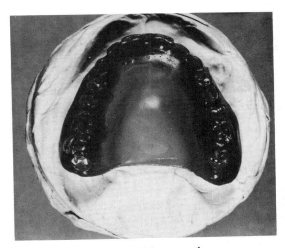

Figure 17.6 A shellac base with wax teeth

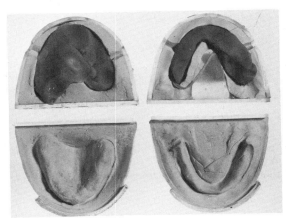

Figure 17.4 Autopolymerizing resin packed into silicone mould

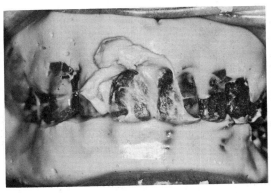

Figure 17.7 Impressions taken in replica dentures together with a centric jaw record

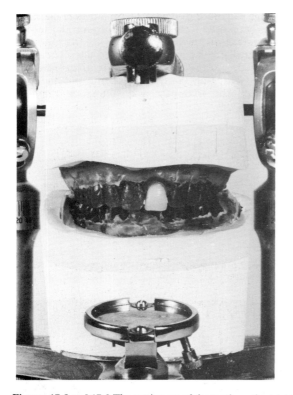
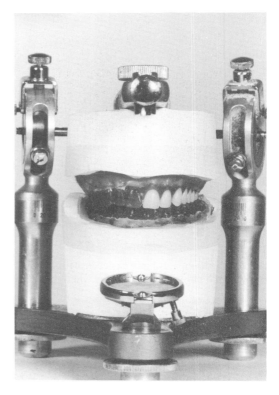

Figures 17.8 and 17.9 The setting-up of the teeth on the trial base

artificial teeth in the same position (Figures 17.8 and 17.9). When all the upper and lower teeth have been set, the try-in can be undertaken, leaving the impression material in place on the base. After a satisfactory try-in the trial dentures can be processed following standard procedures.

Technique 2

After any corrections to the periphery, impressions are taken in the patient's upper and lower dentures in a similar fashion to the procedure used when recording impressions for relining or rebasing complete dentures (Figure 17.10). Also at this clinical stage, an interocclusal wax record is obtained of the occlusal relationship of the dentures and the shade, mould and material of the teeth are recorded; this is particularly important in cases of heavy staining or attrition.

The impressions are poured in dental stone and the casts trimmed in the usual manner. The dentures still on their casts are mounted onto an articulator using the wax occlusal record (Figure 17.11). It is important to use a split mounting technique and a separating medium on the base of the casts to ensure subsequent release of the casts from the articulator

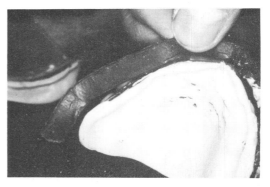

Figure 17.10 Impressions taken in the patient's modified dentures

mounting plaster. Using standard dental laboratory procedures, reversible hydrocolloid duplicating material is used to construct moulds of the dentures on their casts (Figure 17.12). When set the casts and dentures are removed from the mould and the dentures removed from the casts. (The dentures are then cleaned of impression material and returned to the patient.) Sprue holes are cut one in each side leading to the distal aspects of the denture base (Figure 17.13). The casts, which must be water saturated, are then replaced into the moulds. Molten modelling wax (70°C) is then poured down one sprue hole until the mould is filled (Figure 17.14), the other sprue hole allowing for the escape of air. When the wax is hard the wax dentures are removed from the mould. The cast and wax dentures are then replaced onto the articulator where they are relocated on the split mounting plaster (Figure 17.15).

Setting-up with this technique is the same as before; the wax teeth are removed and replaced with artificial teeth. The dentures partially and completely set-up are shown in Figures 17.16 and 17.17. After a satisfactory try-in the dentures are processed in the usual way.

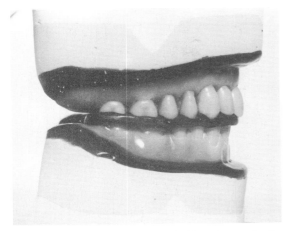

Figure 17.11 The dentures mounted with an interocclusal wax record

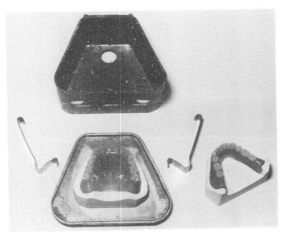

Figure 17.12 Duplication of the dentures using agar-agar moulds

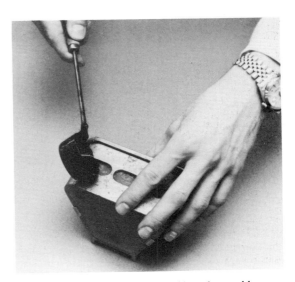

Figure 17.14 The wax being poured into the mould

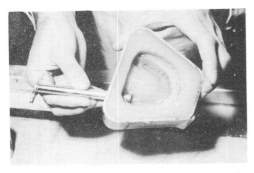

Figure 17.13 Sprue holes cut to allow for the pouring of the wax

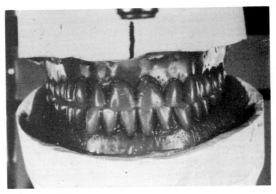

Figure 17.15 Cast and wax dentures re-mounted on the articulator

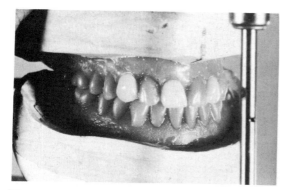

Figure 17.16 A partially completed set-up

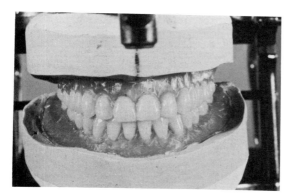

Figure 17.17 A fully completed set-up ready for trial

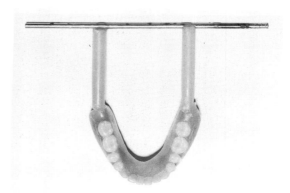

Figure 17.18 Duplication of a patient's denture sprues and wires added

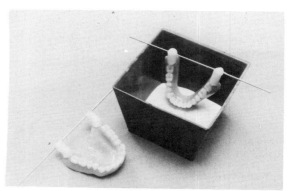

Figure 17.19 Dentures in flask

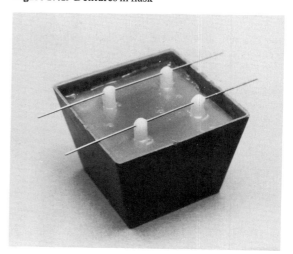

Figure 17.20 Duplicating material fills the flask

Technique 3

This procedure for the construction of replica dentures is well suited in those cases where a precise copy is not required as alterations are needed, but similarity in the denture shape and occlusal plane level is required. The technique is a variation on the previous themes and involves the production of autopolymerizing resin replicas of the dentures that are being worn using a reversible hydrocolloid mould.

The denture periphery is modified and sticky wax, approximately 2 cm in length, is attached to the last molars on the patient's old upper and lower dentures to form sprues. Rigid wire is attached across the sticky wax sprues (Figure 17.18) and the dentures are suspended in a container. To facilitate easy removal of the hydrocolloid from the container and positive relocation when it is replaced, it is important that the sides of the container are tapered outwards from the base to the top, with both the base and top being open. A large nick cut into the bottom of the flask will make the relocation obvious, and the cutting of grooves in the top edges will locate the wire cross pieces (Figure 17.19). The hydrocolloid is poured so as to completely cover the dentures (Figure 17.20).

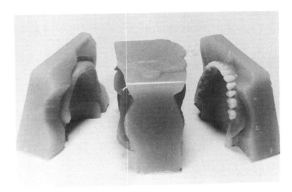

Figure 17.21 Separation of the mould and removal of the dentures

When set the mould is removed from the container, and with a sharp knife, cuts are made along the flanges of the dentures to allow the mould to be separated and to facilitate the removal of the dentures (Figure 17.21). Once the dentures have been removed, the mould is replaced in the container.

Autopolymerizing resin material is mixed to the consistency of a smooth cream and is poured into one sprue hole for the upper and one sprue hole for the lower denture until it extrudes from the opposite sprue hole (Figure 17.22). The resin may be bench cured or cured in a polyclave.

When cured the duplicate dentures are removed from the mould and sprues trimmed off, restoring these dentures to the original shape.

The replica dentures can then be used for taking impressions and, by using an interocclusal wax record, the occlusal relationship can be obtained. Casts are poured into the impressions and the replica dentures are placed onto the articulator using the occlusal registration.

The trial denture is best achieved by removing the upper replica denture from its model, adapting a wax base and setting-up the upper teeth to the replica lower denture and then removing the lower replica denture and setting-up the lower to the upper. Obviously any changes required in setting postions must be observed. Waxing up follows standard procedures and after a satisfactory try-in the dentures are processed to finish in the usual way.

The three techniques described can obviously be varied and adjusted to suit a particular case, the laboratory and clinical time and facilities available, as well as the individual clinician or technician's personal preferences. There are obviously advantages and disadvantages to using any of these copy techniques. The technique of pouring molten wax into a mould often fails to produce sharp detail due to the contraction of the wax. Also, using autopolymerizing resins with a high monomer content

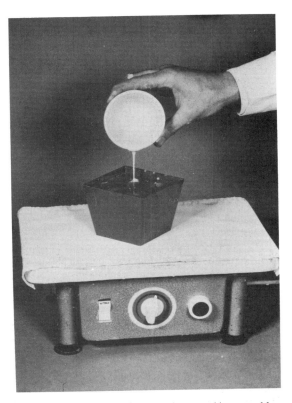

Figure 17.22 Autopolymerizing resin poured into mould

that pour easily into a sprue hole, will create a denture which is not a perfect copy due to the large polymerization contraction. If doughs are packed into a split two-part mould then there is the inevitable risk of incomplete closure and of distortion. Also, when using copy dentures in the mouth to take impressions, it must be remembered that if the dentures are not located *in situ* correctly, then this can give incorrect orientation of the occlusal plane, lip support and centre line.

Overdentures

Overdentures are dentures which are fitted over the rootface of the tooth. Generally, they are complete dentures and the roots are usually endodontically treated and the root canal filled with amalgam, composite or glass ionomer cement (Figure 17.23). A number of roots may be retained in this way thus keeping the alveolar bone intact and aiding retention.

In some cases the tooth may be so worn that it may be retained in its vital state or in some cases a gold coping may be cemented over the tooth.

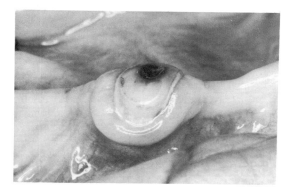

Figure 17.23 A lower canine prepared as support for an overdenture

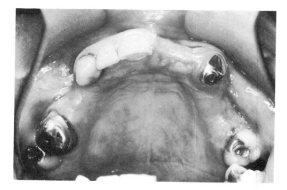

Figure 17.24 An eccentric attachment used as support and retention for a partial denture

The gold copings or, in the case of endodontically treated teeth, a gold diaphragm may be used in conjunction with precision attachments such as that in Figure 17.24. Magnets held in the denture and stainless steel keepers in the teeth may also be used (Figure 17.25). The laboratory procedures for these techniques are complex and beyond the scope of this text and reference should be made to specialized textbooks on this subject.

Where the root of a tooth with a simple gold coping is being used as support the techniques for the construction of complete overdentures are exactly the same as for edentulous patients, but elastic impression materials must be used.

Reciprocal impression technique (neutral zone)

Some patients experience difficulty in wearing complete lower dentures. This is often the case with elderly patients who come to complete denture wearing at a late stage in their life. One of the problems of patients in adapting to dentures is the position of the occlusal plane and the buccolingual position of the artificial teeth. It is important that the tooth position should be such that the tongue and cheeks are able to manipulate food onto the occlusal table and to use these muscular forces as a means of retaining the denture. In order to provide this information to the laboratory on a more scientific basis a technique has been developed to record the neutral zone, or zone of minimal conflict, which is called the reciprocal impression technique. This technique enables the polished surfaces of the denture to be better delineated and also the position of the artificial teeth to be placed in an area of minimal muscular activity. The technique which is generally found to be most suitable is outlined.

Final impressions are taken in the usual manner and the occlusal rims are then made on these casts.

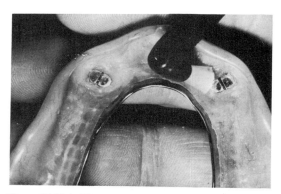

Figure 17.25 A Gillings split magnet used for overdenture retention

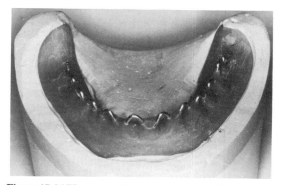

Figure 17.26 The preparation of the base and the retaining wires for the reciprocal impression technique

An autopolymerizing acrylic resin base is then made on the lower cast to which is attached a small metal retaining wire upon which the impression is recorded (Figure 17.26). The reciprocal impression is achieved using an impression material such as silicone putty, which is preferably mixed with half the normal amount of hardening material, thus lengthening the working time. The putty is moulded onto the base plate to the same dimensions as a wax occlusal rim and this is then placed in the patient's mouth and the patient is instructed to (a) open wide, (b) swallow, (c) lick the upper lip, (d) say ooh! (e) say ah! and (f) say eeh! When all these procedures have been carried out (Figure 17.27), the base plate may be removed from the mouth and, with care, the height of the rim reduced to the required occlusal plane. It can then be replaced in the patient's mouth and the muscular activity and final trimming repeated. When the putty has hardened, the jaw record and the impression may be returned to the laboratory.

Laboratory procedure

The jaw record is used to articulate the casts in the usual way and then the reciprocal impression is placed on the lower cast and plaster keys made lingually and buccally on the sides to form a mould (Figure 17.28). The base plate and reciprocal impression may then be removed from the cast and the mould. A new autopolymerizing base, or a wax base with wire strengthener, is then adapted to the cast. The sectional plaster keys are then soaked in

water, or coated with a suitable separator and then placed *in situ* onto the lower model. Wax is then melted in a ladle and poured into the mould through the space between the buccal and lingual sides of the occlusal surface (Figure 17.29).

When the wax is set, the sectional plaster mould is separated and a hard wax reciprocal rim, which is a duplicate of the impression, is reduced to occlude with the upper rim in the centric jaw relationship. Care must be exercised in trimming down the occlusal surface to avoid disturbing the lateral surfaces.

Setting of the teeth

The upper anterior teeth are set first to give the desired lip support and aesthetic requirements. All of the lower teeth are then set, starting with the lower anteriors. This is done while removing just enough wax from the hard wax reciprocal occlusal rim to allow for one tooth to be set at a time. It is important to check with the plaster index that the teeth are set within the confines of the mould (Figure 17.30). If there is a limited space within the confines of the plaster index, it may be necessary to leave off the premolar or even a molar if there is

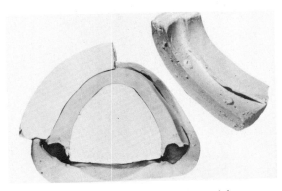

Figure 17.27 Completed reciprocal impression

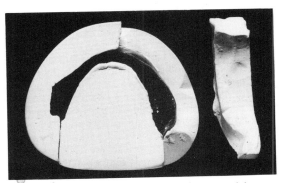

Figure 17.29 The production of a wax duplicate of the reciprocal impression

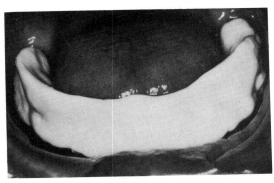

Figure 17.28 Plaster keys are prepared around the reciprocal impression

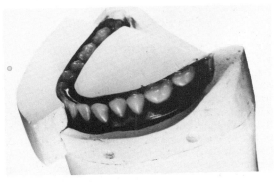

Figure 17.30 The teeth set into the confines of the plaster keys

insufficient space to set all of the teeth. Once all the lower teeth are set, the upper posteriors can be set to give maximum occlusal contact. Adjustment will usually have to be made to the lower teeth and it is important when doing this to ensure that the teeth stay within the confines of the mould.

The upper denture is waxed up for try-in in the usual manner, the lower denture needs no waxing up, it needs only smoothing and trimming around the gingival margins of the teeth. When the trial of the dentures is satisfactorily completed, they are flasked, processed and finished in the usual manner, care being taken with the lower denture to polish it very lightly to avoid losing detail from the surface.

Repairs, additions and relines to existing dentures

Fracture of a denture, or the teeth separating away from the denture base, may be a consequence of a variety of different reasons. Whenever a denture is returned for repair, it is important to ascertain the cause of failure and, if possible, remedy this before effecting the repair.

Causes of fracture may be a consequence of the patient dropping the denture onto the floor during cleaning procedures, and the patient should be advised to always clean the denture over a water-filled wash basin to prevent further accidents.

If upper posterior teeth are set too far buccally to the crest of the ridge, then masticatory loads will transmit a flexing component to the mid-line and this, coupled with a deep frenal notch which leads to stress concentration, may result in denture fracture. Poor laboratory processing procedures may also lead to denture failure; teeth separating from the denture base at their interface are often a consequence of inadequate wax removal. A poor fitting denture and dentures that have endured heavy occlusal wear are also reasons for denture failure. Whatever the reason, it should be established and a remedy sought if a further occurrence is to be avoided.

Repair of acrylic complete dentures

The parts of the denture must be reassembled accurately and sealed together on their polished surfaces with sticky wax. It is necessary to strengthen the sticky wax bond still further by the addition of some support across the arch; a piece of wire or metal or match may be used for this purpose. A plaster-of-Paris cast is poured into the fitting surface of the denture and, when this has set, the broken parts of the denture are removed from the cast. The edges of the fracture line are prepared by grinding with a handpiece and stone so that there is a space of

about 5 mm between the edges which should be tapered as shown in Figure 17.31. These trimmed surfaces are then polished with pumice. The cast is coated with a separator and the sections of the denture are placed onto the cast (Figure 17.32).

Most repairs are undertaken using autopolymerizing acrylic resin. The strength of these resins is inferior to that of the heat-cured resins. However, they are generally preferred because they are easier and much quicker to use than heated cured systems. When heat-cured materials are used to effect a denture repair, the prepared repair surface is waxed up to its normal original contour and the denture is flasked using the hooded method so that only the wax surface is exposed. The processing procedures are then the same as those described in Chapter 14. If a palate is to be replaced, or any other large area, then a heat-cured repair is preferred.

When dentures are repaired using the autopolymerizing resins, the resin is mixed with a free flowing fluid consistency (ratio 2:1 volume) and the mix is flowed onto the surfaces of the join to slight excess. The denture *in situ* on the cast is then placed into a hydroflask with a water temperature of about 35°C and a pressure of 2.2 bar. It is left in the hydroflask for approximately 30 minutes. The repaired denture is then removed from the cast and trimmed and polished in the normal manner.

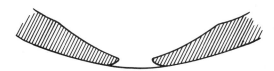

Figure 17.31 Preparation of a fractured denture

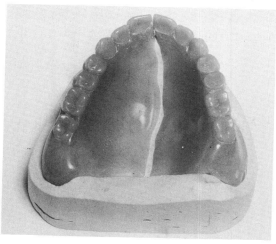

Figure 17.32 The fractured denture placed on the cast prior to repair

Tooth replacement

The cast is poured into the fitting surface of the denture. If the displaced tooth is available and is undamaged, it is repositioned on the denture base and secured with sticky wax. If a new tooth is to be used, the denture base is shaped to accept it. The tooth is held in position with wax which is contoured to the shape of the denture base.

A plaster matrix is formed to the labial surface of the tooth and the adjacent teeth to supply a locating key (Figure 17.33). The wax is flushed away. The ridge lap surface of the tooth is prepared with mechanical retention. The lingual or palatal surface of the denture base is trimmed away to develop a space for the repair material. Both prepared surfaces are polished with pumice. The labial gingival surface is, if possible, left untouched so that the repair is essentially invisible.

The denture, tooth, matrix and cast are assembled and the autopolymerizing resin introduced into the palatal or lingual space. After polymerization in a hydroflask the repair is trimmed and polished.

The loss of a number of teeth, or, in some cases, only one tooth, may necessitate a cast of the opposing dentition or denture be used to help with the articulation.

Adding a tooth to a denture as an immediate replacement

Should it be necessary to add a tooth to the denture as an immediate replacement, then this procedure is similar to that described in the previous section. The stone tooth to be replaced is removed from the cast, the socket prepared, and a suitable stock tooth ground and fitted to the socket (Figure 17.34). This tooth is then waxed to the remaining part of the denture and a plaster matrix is made. If autopolymerizing acrylic resins are to be used the wax is flushed away but if heat-cured resins are to be used, the denture is flasked and packed in the manner described earlier. If a tooth, or teeth, has already been extracted and needs to be added to the existing denture, an impression is taken of the patient's mouth with the denture in place, as previously but, in addition, an impression of the lower opposing dentition will be required in order to articulate the two casts prior to waxing up the new teeth on the master cast (Figure 17.34). When the new artifical

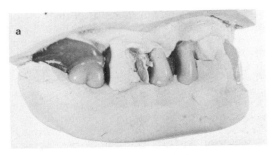
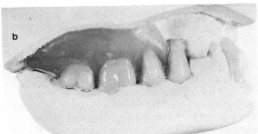

Figure 17.34 The addition of an immediate tooth to a denture. (a) Before removal of tooth. (b) New tooth waxed into position

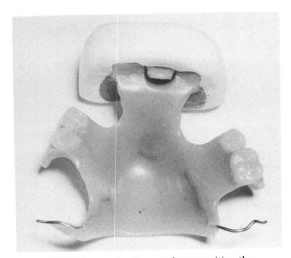

Figure 17.33 The locating key used to reposition the artificial teeth

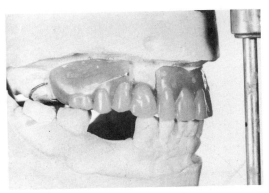

Figure 17.35 Mounted casts to ensure the correct articulation of the replaced tooth

teeth have been waxed into position and joined to the old plastic denture base, it can be flasked in exactly the same way as described for a repair, or a plastic matrix may again be made of the teeth, wax flushed away and an autopolymerizing acrylic resin flown into the voids. With either technique, once the acrylic resin has been added and processed, the dentures are trimmed and polished in the usual way.

Repairs and additions to metal dentures

An impression of the mouth is taken with the denture *in situ*. Should it be necessary to add metal parts, such as clasps or occlusal rests, by soldering to the existing denture base, then the acrylic resin parts must be removed. Before removal of the saddles, the cast is coated with a separating medium and an index poured in plaster of Paris (Figure 17.36). The index and the cast, if required, may be fixed to the upper and lower arms respectively of an articulator. If the teeth to be added are already extracted, an impression of the opposing jaw should be taken and articulated on a movable articulator with a master cast containing the denture.

If clasps, etc. are to be added from wrought material they may be soldered to the base as described on page 95. The new part to be added may however need to be cast using the same technique as describe in Chapter 12. When the new part has been polished, it can be seated on the cast and soldered in the same way as a wrought wire. Once the denture base has been completed it is polished as if it were a new metal denture and seated on the cast.

With both gold and cobalt–chromium denture bases, the acrylic parts can now be replaced. A major part of the resin holding the teeth to the base is removed and the teeth waxed back into position by reference to the plaster index or to the cast of the opposing jaw. When flasked, like a new partial

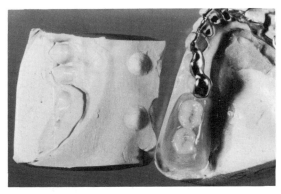

Figure 17.36 The use of an index to locate the artifical teeth prior to removal of the acrylic base

denture, and the wax replaced by acrylic resin, the occlusion of the repaired denture should require the minimum of adjustment

Relines of complete and partial dentures

Relining of dentures only modifies the impression surface of dentures. Its objective is to improve the stability of the dentures by restoring the fit. There must be no change in the vertical dimension. The clinical technique for relining complete and partial dentures involves removing the undercuts from the fitting surface of the denture base and registering an impression in the base using an impression material, such as zinc oxide paste, Korrecta wax or silicone elastomeric impression material.

Partial dentures

A new impression is then cast and must include, in the case of the partial denture, the metal framework. All plastic partial dentures are difficult to reline satisfactorily and a new partial denture is more easily made. The denture is removed from the cast and the impression material is eliminated.

A simple technique that may be used with metal partial dentures is to remove a thin film of acrylic resin from all over the saddle area and coat the cast with a separating material. A thin mix of auto-polymerizing acrylic resin denture base material is coated on the fitting surface of the denture, which is then seated carefully on the cast. The metal framework is pressed firmly into position. It is then placed into a hydroflask with a water temperature of about 35°C and a pressure of 2.2 bar. It is left in the hydroflask for approximately 30 minutes. The relined denture can then be trimmed and polished.

The localization of the metal base is often difficult and, in this situation, an index is prepared prior to removal of the impression material and the cast and index fixed into a frame (Figure 17.37). The technique is then the same as before, since the frame and index maintain the denture in the correct relationship to the cast and this fits inside the hydroflask. This technique, using an autopolymeriz-ing acrylic resin, is more accurate than the more conventional techniques.

The conventional method of relining a partial denture of this type is to prepare a cast as for the self-curing technique, together with the necessary index. The denture is then removed from the cast and a large part of the acrylic resin, bonding the teeth to the metal work, is removed and the teeth fixed into the index (Figure 17.37). The denture is then waxed-up, as in the usual procedure of setting up the partial denture. When complete, it is flasked and packed in exactly the same way as if it were a

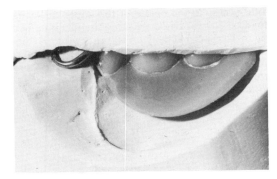

Figure 17.37 A partial denture mounted on a localizing frame for the relining procedure

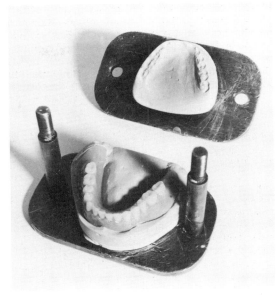

Figure 17.38 A complete denture prepared for relining

new denture. In some cases, the stone cast on which the denture was constructed may be available when a corrected cast technique may be used (see page 99). In this case the cast, when poured, must be articulated with an index and treated as above.

Complete dentures

The impression in the denture, when received in the laboratory, should be beaded before being poured. The undersurface of the cast is then scored and it is mounted onto the lower arm of a simple hinge articulator or, alternatively, a jig specifically designed for use when relining dentures can be employed.

An overbite is poured in plaster. It must contact the occlusal surfaces and incisal edges of the teeth, as well as their palatal or lingual surface. It must also touch the posterior projection of the cast. The upper arm of the articulator, or upper member of the reline jig is embedded in the plaster ensuring that they contact their stops to maintain the relationship between the overbite and cast once the denture is removed. The overbite is trimmed to expose the buccal and labial surfaces of the teeth: it must be possible to observe the fit of the occlusal surface and incisal edges of the teeth in the overbite.

Once the plaster has set, the articulator or jig is opened and the denture is removed from the cast (Figure 17.38). The impression material is removed from the denture and from the cast. The impression surface and borders of the denture are reduced by 1–2 mm using a stone and handpiece. The fitting surface and borders of the dentures are polished with pumice.

Sodium alginate separating solution is painted onto the surfaces of the cast. In upper denture relines the post-dam should be carved before the sodium alginate is applied. The denture is accurately seated in the overbite and retained in the correct position by the use of sticky wax.

When autopolymerizing resins are used to reline the denture, the material is mixed and placed into the sulcus areas of the cast and over the fitting surface of the denture. An excess of resin is applied. When the material is at a very soft dough stage, the overbite and cast are gently brought together, the correct relationship of overbite to cast must be checked by preserving contact between their respective posterior regions and the locating stops on the reline jig or the stop screw on the articulator. The excess material will extrude out and must be trimmed away.

With the denture *in situ* on the cast and the mounting jig securely fixed, the whole is placed into a hydroflask with a water temperature of about 35°C and a pressure of 2.2 bar. It is left in the hydroflask for approximately 30 minutes. The relined denture is then removed from the cast and trimmed and polished in the normal manner. Often, it is necessary to rebase complete dentures. This technique is more appropriate than relining when labial flanges or new palates are required for the dentures.

The preparation of the denture and the impression techniques are as described for relines. When the denture is separated from the cast and the impression material removed from the dentures, in the case of an upper denture, the palate is removed to within 5 mm of the teeth and the acrylic on the labial and buccal aspect is cut away around the necks of the teeth. The cut surfaces are then smoothed with pumice to make the junction between old and new resin less obvious. The horseshoe of teeth, which is held together by the old acrylic, is then accurately seated into the overbite and retained *in situ* by sticky wax. The overbite and cast are now related to each other by means of their mounting jigs or articulator and wax is flowed between the cast and the surfaces of the denture. The wax is built up and then the overbite is separated from the teeth to permit access to the palate of the upper or lingual side of the lower. These areas are then built up with wax in the normal way. The wax work is then trimmed in the same way as it would be for a complete denture set-up. After waxing-up is completed, the dentures are flasked, processed and finished in the usual way.

Appendix I

Removable partial dentures

Guide to examination and planning

(1) Main complaint or desire.

(2) Previous and present medical history. Social history.

(3) Dental and denture experience.

(4) General examination of the face.

(5) Examination of present dentures.

(6) Charting: according to the three sections of the separate sheet.

(7) Examination of the mouth:
Lips, cheeks, tongue and floor of mouth, hard and soft palates, ridges, tuberosity and retromolar areas.

(8) Examination of occlusion:
Vertical dimension.
Natural occlusal stops.
Premature contacts and slides.
Contact in lateral and protrusive excursions.
Masticatory efficiency assessment (subjective).

(9) Accessory information:
Radiographs.
Surveyed study casts mounted in centric occlusion.
Oral hygiene performance and diet.

(10) Patient's attitudes to:
Preventative advice.
Appearance and condition of own natural teeth.

(11) Prognosis of natural dentition with respect to:
Caries. Stability of the teeth in occlusion.
Loading of the teeth and the opposing denture.

(12) Primary treatment plan:
Oral hygiene and dietary advice.
Restoration with or without partial denture?
Preliminary denture design.
Conservation and restorative plan.
Occlusal adjustment.

(13) Denture treatment:
Control of oral hygiene and periodontal conditions.
Final denture design.
Tooth preparations.

Figure I.1 gives a typical chart to be filled in with patient's medical history and details of examination of the teeth.

134

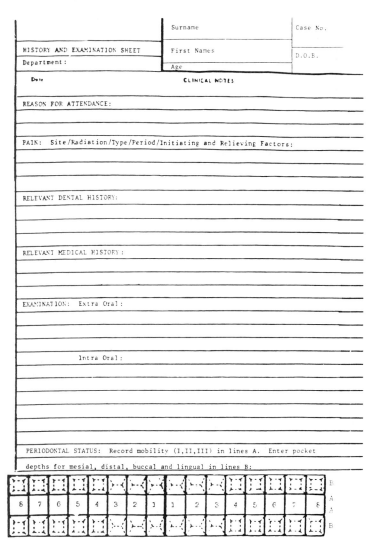

Figure I.1 Patient chart for taking medical history and details of examination of teeth

RESTORATION AND CAVITY CHART (from CLINICAL examination): Enter cavities, restorations, spaces, etc. in lines X and other details (partial eruptions, gold, etc.) in lines Y:

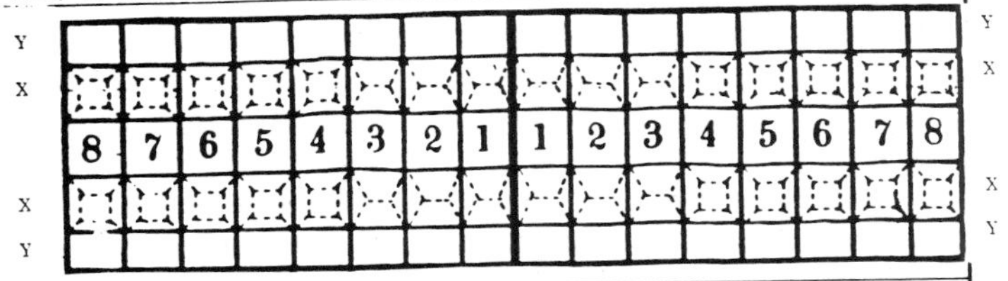

Y																Y
X																X
	8	7	6	5	4	3	2	1	1	2	3	4	5	6	7	8
X																X
Y																Y

Staff Initials:

EXAMINATION OF OCCLUSION:

RADIOGRAPHIC FINDINGS:
Caries:

Other:

SPECIAL EXAMINATIONS:

CONDITIONS DIAGNOSED:

PROJECTED RESTORATIONS: Enter design in lines X and material in lines Y:

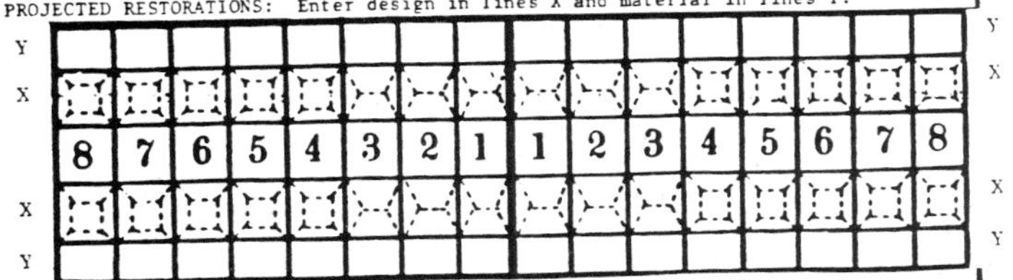

Y																Y
X																X
	8	7	6	5	4	3	2	1	1	2	3	4	5	6	7	8
X																X
Y																Y

Signatures: Undergraduate: Staff:

Figure I.1 (*cont.*)

Appendix II

Methods of assessing the periodontal condition and the amount of plaque on teeth

Russell Periodontal Index (PI)

Each tooth is scored and the whole mouth summated and divided by the teeth used. The mean value will be between 0 and 8.

0 –Negative: There is neither overt inflammation in the investing tissues nor loss of function due to destruction of supporting tissues.
1 –Mild gingivitis: There is an overt area of inflammation in the free gingivae, but this area does not circumscribe the tooth.
2 –Gingivitis: Inflammation completely circumscribes the tooth, but there is no apparent break in the epithelial attachment.
6 –Gingivitis with pocket formation: The epithelial attachment has been broken and there is a pocket (not merely a deepened gingival crevice due to swelling in the free gingiva). There is no interference with normal masticatory function, the tooth is firm in its socket and has not drifted, horizontal bone loss is less than half the length of the root.
8 –Advanced destruction with loss of masticatory function: The tooth may be lost, may have drifted, may sound dull on percussion with a metallic instrument, may be depressible in its socket. More than half the tooth root has advanced bone loss and a definite bony pocket with widening of the periodontal membrane.

Debris Index (Green and Vermillion, 1964)

Stain plaque with erythrocin.

Plaque scores:

0 –No visible plaque.
1 –< third of tooth surface covered.
2 –> half, < two-thirds of tooth surface covered.
3 –> two-thirds of tooth surface covered.

Select six surfaces from four posterior and two anterior teeth. Add score and divide by 6.

Preferred teeth:

Buccal upper first molars.
Lingual lower first molars.
Labial of upper right central incisor.
Labial of lower left central incisor.

When teeth are missing adaptation is required.

Appendix III

Complete dentures

Guide to examination and planning

(1) Main complaint or desire.
Previous and present medical and social history.
(2) Dental and denture experiences.
(3) The face:
Build, complexion, skin, angles of lips, profile and face height.
Appearance and character of dentures.
(4) Examination of mouth:
Inflammation of mucosa or lesions.
Saliva and wetness of mucosa.
Appearance of tongue.
Denture-bearing area – palate and vibrating line, floor of mouth, mylohyoid ridge, tuberosities, retromolar pads.
Size, shape, consistency and relationship of ridges.
Cheeks and lips, including muscle tone and activity.
(5) Occlusion of present dentures:
Vertical dimension.
Tooth material and wear.
Initial contact in centric relation.
Relationship with clenching.
Contact in lateral and protrusive excursions.
Patient's assessment of masticatory efficiency.

(6) Examination of present dentures:
Retention and extension of bases – labial, buccal and lingual borders, frena, mylohyoid ridges, retromolar pads, posterior palate, hambular notches.
Stability and fit.
(7) Accessory information:
Radiographs.
Microbiological culture.
Haemoglobin assessment.
(8) Patient's personality and expectations.
(9) Treatment plan:
Conditioning reline of present dentures.
Treatment of denture stomatitis.
Occlusal correction of present dentures.
Copy of present dentures?
Impression trays and materials.
Registration of neutral zone.
Occlusal vertical dimension the same or changed?
Tooth selection and positions (anterior and posterior) the same or changed?
Advice on denture wearing and cleaning, denture limitations and nutrition.
(10) Prognosis of denture treatment with respect to:
Main complaint or desire of patient.
Anatomical or physiological difficulties of the mouth.
Appearance and function.

Appendix IV

Surveying

If part of the denture enters an undercut area relative to its insertion path, the denture will not be capable of being properly seated in the mouth. The procedure of locating and delineating the contours of the teeth and soft tissue to ascertain these undercut areas is one of the principal reasons for surveying. These areas can then be eliminated and the technique for carrying this out is described in the appropriate chapter.

The process of surveying is carried out on an instrument, similar to that shown in Figure IV.1. The majority of surveyors possess a double-jointed arm, at the end of which is a vertical rod which can thus be moved in a variety of positions on a horizontal plane. At the bottom of the vertical rod is a chuck which will hold an analysing rod, pencil lead, undercut gauges or chisels, as may be required (Figure IV.2). The purposes of surveying are:

(1) To determine the most acceptable path of insertion and removal, which is undertaken by placing an analysing rod in the holder and attaching the cast to the movable table. If the rod is then brought down to the convex surfaces of the teeth on the cast it will be seen that spaces occur above and below the contact between the stone cast and the rod (Figure IV.3). This point of contact represents the greatest convexity of the tooth, and when all such points are joined together a line is formed around the tooth which is called the survey line. Tilting the cast on the table will cause the line to move from one position to another. Areas below the survey line are called undercut areas, or areas of gingival convergence and those above the survey lines are called areas of occlusal convergence or non-undercut areas. By tilting the cast on the table it is possible to decide which is the best

path of insertion and removal of the denture for that particular area.

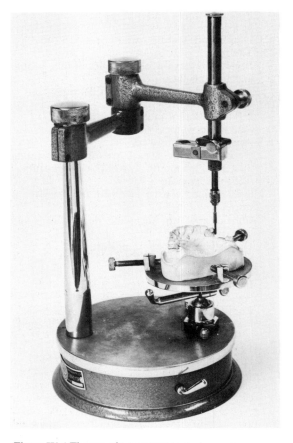

Figure IV.1 The use of a surveyor to study a cast

138

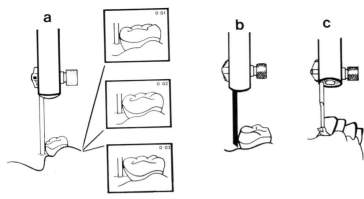

Figure IV.2 Various instruments which can be used in the surveyor: (a) undercut gauges, (b) carbon marker, (c) wax trimmer

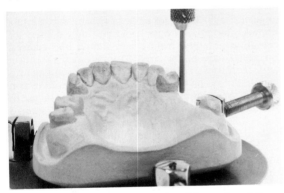

Figure IV.3 Illustrates the convexity of the tooth and the survey line

(2) The insertion and removal of the denture is controlled by the proximal tooth surfaces and these surfaces are called guide planes. To reduce the problem to simple terms, the lateral outline of a single edentulous space must be considered. If the saddle of the denture fills this edentulous space exactly, as a cube fits into a box, it will be evident that there is only one path of displacement by which the saddle can be removed (Figure IV.4). Many shapes of saddle exist and the aim of surveying is to plan the tilt of the cast and make the necessary preparations in the mouth so that the guiding planes of the teeth will allow the saddle to be displaced in one path only. For instance, consider a saddle similar to the shape in Figure IV.5. It will be seen that if it is surveyed with the occlusal plane placed horizontally, the undercut areas are distributed evenly on both sides of the abutment teeth. The saddle will then pass in and out in one direction. Should the cast be tilted, however, to arrange the undercut at one end various paths of displacement are possible and the saddle can be rotated easily out of position.

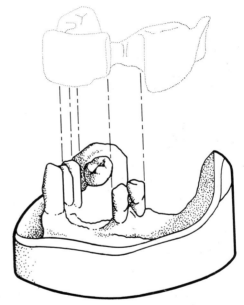

Figure IV.4 Parallel-sided saddles can only be removed in one direction

Working on a similar premise, all the various types of saddle areas can be examined and the cast should also be viewed in a coronal plane since the lingual surfaces of the teeth form the sides of a large saddle when the connectors join the parts together. In the upper jaw, in a coronal plane, a typical open type of saddle similar to Figure IV.6d usually occurs with many paths of displacement. If the denture can be confined to one path of displacement, then positive clasp action will retain the denture in place. Once the path of insertion has been decided, a carbon pencil is placed in the surveyor and the contours of the teeth and soft tissues are marked.

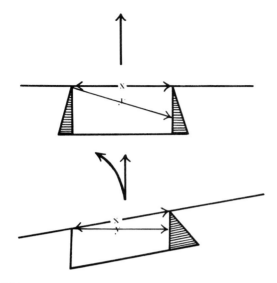

Figure IV.5 Tilted cast to show various paths of displacement

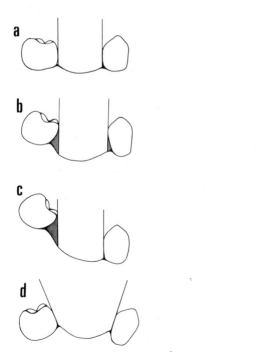

Figure IV.6 (a–c) Various saddle shapes; (d) palatal view of a denture showing lack of guiding planes and an 'open' type of saddle

(3) The location and measurement of the areas on the teeth which may be used for retention can also be undertaken using the undercut gauges in the surveyor. In those areas where clasps are to

be placed, the appropriate size of undercut gauge can be used and the points marked on the stone cast.

In selecting a path of insertion certain factors have to be taken into account. First, the tilt of the cast on the surveyor will affect the position of the survey line and in the upper and lower anterior regions of the mouth it is better to position clasps as near the gingival margins of the teeth as possible. Aesthetics is therefore a factor which must be considered when finalizing the path of insertion.

Similarly, when anterior teeth are being replaced, where undercuts exist on the abutment teeth adjacent to the edentulous areas, an unaesthetic space between the artificial and the natural teeth will occur and it is therefore better to tilt the cast even when it is to the detriment of the factors already discussed. Second, as the tips of clasp arms engage the undercut areas on the teeth to predetermined amounts, where possible the degree of retention obtained from clasps should be balanced on either side of the arch to give equal retention and, therefore, a provision of a buccal retaining arm should always be balanced by a buccal retaining arm on the opposite side of the jaw. This helps to prevent displacement along any but the planned path. Similar types of clasps on each side of the arch should engage the same amount of undercut, but if clasps of different materials are used the undercut must be adjusted to give the same degree of retention.

To summarize, therefore, it will be seen that those factors to be taken into account when surveying are:

(1) The selection of the path of insertion and removal and the provision of guiding planes.
(2) The detection and elimination of interference with the path of insertion.
(3) The selection of the best type of clasps for a given situation to give the correct amount of retention.
(4) The achievement of an aesthetic result.

Recording the path of insertion

Having obtained the desired tilt on the cast, three points are marked on the cast near distinctive anatomical points in the same horizontal plane. This is done by allowing the pencil to rise to its highest position and, if possible, locking it so that it will not move downwards. The tip of the pencil is now free to move in only one horizontal plane and will mark this plane on the cast (Figure 12.1). Provided it passes through anatomical points, any cast can be re-orientated to this position by placing the same anatomical landmarks in a horizontal plane.

Appendix V

Retention of complete dentures

Retention of complete upper dentures in the first instance is dependent upon the physical forces created by the presence of a film of saliva between the denture and the tissues. Since the lower jaw is mobile and the tissue available much smaller, the physical forces on the lower denture are minimal and retention is dependent on the muscles of the cheeks and tongue holding the denture in place.

Retention in complete upper dentures

It must be remembered that dentures are in a dynamic state since they are stressed on soft foundations and during function must move about; this is particularly so during mastication.

Stefan (1874) suggested the formula for the movement of two plates away from each other

$$\frac{dH}{dt} = \frac{2FH^3}{3Va^2}$$

where V is the viscosity, a is the area of the plates, F is the force of separation and H is the interplate distance. Integration of this with respect to time gives the following formula

$$t = \frac{3Va^2}{4F} \left[\frac{1}{H_1^2} - \frac{1}{H_2^2} \right]$$

and if H_2 is large compared with H_1^2 it can be discounted, leaving a formula

$$Ft - \frac{3Va^2}{4} \left[\frac{1}{H_1^2} \right]$$

We can therefore see that denture retention is related to time and the displacing force. It is possible to unseat a denture if the force is high in a short time or if the force is low over a longer period. This is experimentally provable and has been shown to be so. Also work has shown that retention is directly related to viscosity.

From this formula, we cannot therefore say that dentures will have maximum retention when the area of the denture is as large as possible and has intimate contact with the soft tissues with the thinnest possible film of saliva and where the saliva has a relatively high viscosity. The accuracy of the impression is thus important and also that it should be correctly extended.

In the mouth, under function, the denture must be completely wet and be covered by a salivary film; it is equivalent to two glass plates under water. Surface tension is thus not a factor in denture retention, and adhesion and cohesion, whilst having some effect, are primarily important in providing the physical property of viscosity of the fluid film and its ability to flow over the surfaces of the tissues and the denture.

It has been suggested that the wettability of the material will be of importance and that a factor $\cos \theta$ of the contact angle should be included in the formula. However, since the denture within a few minutes of being within the oral cavity will be covered in a salivary pellicle of mucopolysaccharide, it is the relationship between the salivary film and the pellicle that is important. The contact angle, in this case, is so low that $\cos \theta$ approximates to 1; thus the inclusion of this factor in the formula would be of no value. No clinical evidence has been produced to show that surface tension or the wettability of the denture is important. Roydhouse (1960) and Barbenel (1971) support the view inherent in the

Stefan equation that restriction of flow of saliva will aid retention and this has been experimentally demonstrated by Kawazoe and Hamada (1978). Some discussion still exists, however, as to whether the area involved is the actual area of the denture or the projected area of the denture. Brill (1967) has elaborated upon these principles and produced a formula which expresses the view more simply (see Figure V.1).

$$M = \frac{b \cdot \Delta p \cdot h^2}{12 \cdot l \cdot \eta}$$

In this formula M is the fluid flow in unit time and is proportional to B the length of the slit at right angles to the direction of flow, whilst P is the pressure difference between the oral surface and the palatal surface created by the displacement of the denture, and H is the intervening space between the denture and the tissues. Likewise, it is inversely proportional to L, which is the length of the buccal flange and η is the viscosity.

In order to restrict flow of saliva and give maximum retention therefore, flange height must be as great as possible and the viscosity high, whilst the periphery B must be as long as possible and the contact between the denture and the tissues as small as possible, reducing the salivary film to a minimum. Brill relates this to a piston as in Figure V.2 where it is obvious that of the two figures one (A) will require less force for removal than the other (B).

The direct utilization of muscle forces to increase retention also acts indirectly. Since the tongue, cheeks and lips are pressed against the denture, the slit between the denture and the soft tissues is reduced to a minimum impeding the flow of saliva. Moreover, the contact area between the mucosa and the denture may also be increased, thus increasing the effective area of interfacial seal (Figure V.3).

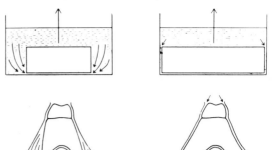

Figure V.2 Diagram to show the effect of a large salivary film and a small salivary film. In A there is a wide slit between the plate and the walls of the vessel. Below there is, similarly, a wide slit between the denture and adjacent structures. In B the slits are narrow

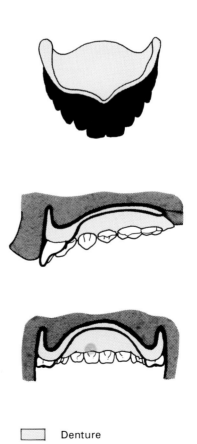

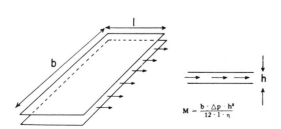

Figure V.1 Diagram representing the denture and the tissues on the flange of a denture (redrawn from Jorgensen, 1959)

| Denture |
| Salivary film |

Figure V.3 The peripheral seal in a complete denture

Retention of the mandibular denture

It is important that dentures are designed to utilize to a maximum the effect of the interfacial seal, particularly in the initial period of denture wearing, since it is during this period that the patient learns to become adjusted to the dentures.

However, with time there will be bone resorption and changes in the tissues such that the effect of the salivary film will be reduced. It is therefore important that the patient learns to develop muscular control of the dentures and this particular-ly applies in the lower jaw. Retention of the lower denture is dependent largely on muscle forces and it can be demonstrated that the retentiveness of the dentures will decrease when the surfaces of the mucous membrane are anaesthetized.

Whilst the retention of the mandibular denture will be primarily due to muscle activity, if the denture is correctly adapted to the tissues and the soft tissues are adapted to the buccal and lingual surfaces, some physical retention should be possible.

Appendix VI

Advice to patients wearing dentures

Now that you have your new dentures there are several things you will want to know about them. At first, they may seem bulky and awkward, and you may find difficulty in controlling them while eating, speaking and swallowing. Do not let these things discourage you however, for they are literally 'teething troubles'. In a week or so the strangeness will wear off and you will not notice the dentures in your mouth; sucking boiled sweets often helps people with new dentures to get accustomed to them. You must train your mouth to use them for eating, as you would have to train your hands to use tools in acquiring a manual skill. Your tongue and cheeks must learn how to control the dentures as you eat. Try to get you tongue on top of the lower denture and take small mouthfuls of food at a time – do not be upset if food and dentures get mixed up at first. Initially, this will require real effort, but soon it will happen automatically. The secret lies in patient perseverance. Some people take weeks or even months to master their dentures – but they find the effort fully rewarded.

Partial dentures are usually less of a problem since they may be attached to the natural teeth but it may still take some time to become adjusted to them.

Dentures should not be worn at night and this is particularly important with partial dentures where retained plaque can cause periodontal disease and caries. There is, however, one exception which is complete immediate dentures, where for the first 3 months they should be cleaned and worn during the night.

Cleaning dentures

Complete dentures

Keep your dentures really clean – rinse them after meals if possible and certainly clean them morning and night. A soft brush and soapy water is best for this purpose. If the teeth get stained a commercially produced cleanser will restore them. *Do not put plastic dentures in hot water, domestic cleaners or antiseptics,* as they will be warped or spoiled in these circumstances. When not in use keep them in clean, cold water.

The best type of cleanser for acrylic resin dentures is a hypochlorite material such as Dentural, but other materials such as Milton which is used to sterilize baby-feeding bottles may be used. Dilute hydrochloric acid cleansers can also be used. Whilst any of the other proprietary materials can be used they are less effective in removing stains and, more importantly, in killing bacteria which lead to candidiasis.

Partial dentures

If the dentures are plastic the method of cleaning is the same as for complete dentures but if metal is present the hypochlorite cleansers must be stabilized. Commercial materials will state that no damage to metal should occur. Chlorine attacks metal and care must be taken to see that the high polish on the metal is not lost. Therefore, generally, hydrochloric acid cleansers are not satisfactory.

Initially the denture should be cleaned carefully with a toothbrush to get into all the crevices and the inside of clasps are best cleaned with a small 'bottle' brush or an interproximal brush designed for the teeth. When all the visible plaque is removed a soaking in the proprietary oxidizing-type cleanser can be employed (i.e. Steradent).

Aftercare

Once the denture has been adjusted and the initial soreness has passed off the dentures should be

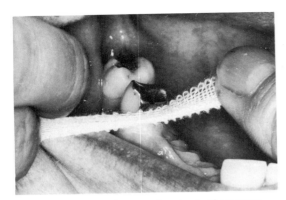

Figure VI.1 The use of tape to clean teeth where space exists

perfectly comfortable and soreness will soon be forgotten. However, should soreness persist you must return for further adjustments. Your mouth changes continually and in the case of complete dentures a yearly review by your dentist is advisable.

In the case of partial dentures this is a more complicated situation. First it is essential to clean your teeth with a fluoride-containing toothpaste after breakfast and last thing at night and also after your midday meal if possible. The use of floss regularly can also be of considerable help in reducing plaque. Between spaced teeth where a large gap exists into which a denture fits, tape is the better material to clean the surface of the teeth (Figure VI.1). This is particularly important around the teeth which touch the denture but all dentures increase the risk of accumulating plaque.

To ensure that your plaque control is satisfactory it is preferable for you to visit a dental hygienist every 3 months and to be seen by your dentist every 6 months. Do not remove partial dentures by pushing under the clasps with your finger nails as this will cause them to bend. It is preferable to grip the plastic holding the artificial teeth between the fingers and lift the denture.

Appendix VII

Safety in the dental laboratory

Safety in the dental laboratory is the responsibility of everyone concerned with that laboratory. Employers have a statutory responsibility, but all technicians and ancillaries working in these laboratories have a need to adopt patterns of activity that are sensible and safe. This requirement extends to a need to work safely and cleanly.

Inhalation protection

There is a risk in all laboratories from the inhalation of dust, toxic fumes and chemicals. It is essential that the machinery used for grinding, polishing, burning out, and monomer handling should be fitted with appropriate dust covers and extractor systems so that dust may be collected and chemical fumes vented away from the workplace. When working with any machinery that generates dust it is essential that the operator wears a facemask.

Dust control devices for specific procedures will only provide satisfactory control if the workplace is maintained in a tidy and clean condition and so good housekeeping is essential. Movement of people through a 'dusty' laboratory area will generate more dust contamination of the area, which may be inhaled. Thus, dust sources such as pumice troughs, plaster of Paris, dental stones, investment materials and sandblasting materials should be controlled by appropriate procedures and storage.

Toxic fumes arise when patterns are being burnt out in the production of metal castings and also when ultrasonic cleaning units are used. The fumes contain ammonia and are unpleasant. The burning out should always be carried out in a well-ventilated room with fume extraction systems, and ultrasonic cleaning units positioned in fume cupboards.

Monomer is a toxic inhalation hazard that is present when dental acrylics are being prepared for packing in the production of a denture or special impression trays. These procedures should, therefore, always be carried out in a fume cupboard with an extraction system. The room should be well ventilated. Airborne monomer may also be produced when acrylic items are ground in finishing procedures. Such grinding should only take place at a bench where there is an extraction system and an appropriate filter in the system.

Eye protection

Eye injury is potentially one of the most serious accidents that may occur in the dental laboratory. There are many procedures which may cause this and a 'minor' injury may easily progress to a more serious state that could involve the loss of the eye.

The dental technician is at risk when working at the bench grinding any hard substance, and high speed grinders for cutting and grinding of dental alloys may be specially dangerous to the operator. Use of irritant and corrosive solutions, as in ultrasonic cleaning baths, also constitute an eye injury hazard.

It is essential that spectacles, visors or faceshields, as appropriate, are worn for all grinding procedures and in procedures involving irritant solutions. Most of the machinery is provided with protective shields behind which the grinding may take place, but particles can easily escape from behind these shields and so individual protection is essential. The protection chosen should conform to the appropriate British Standard for this equipment and it is essential to ensure that the eye protection is suitable for the individual and suitable for the work.

It is sometimes necessary to use prescription safety spectacles and in this case it is essential to ensure that such lenses are suitable for the work being carried out. With some high speed grinding work the prescription spectacles may need to be supplemented by a face visor. All eye protection should have side pieces to protect the sides of the eyes.

It is essential that all technicians understand that they have a responsibility to wear eye or face protection.

Dust masks and goggles can be obtained from Martindale Protection Ltd, Neasdon Lane, London NW10 1RN and face visors from Pul Safe, Safety Products Ltd, Redhill, Surrey.

Protective clothing

Satisfactory protective clothing should always be worn in the dental laboratory. Traditionally, coats or overalls in white are used. They should be comfortable and cover to the neck so that debris is not deposited onto clothing worn underneath. Shoes should be chosen that are satisfactory and safe for the floor coverings of the laboratory. There must be an adequate heel area on the shoes and they should be safe in a situation when a floor may become wet.

Head protection is not usually required in the dental laboratory, although hair protection is necessary. Hair should be short, or tied back at all times because of the risk from rotating machinery and fire risk from bunsen burners.

Skin and clothing may be damaged by corrosive solutions. Protective heavy-duty gloves are necessary when using some sandblasting machines.

Fire protection

The laboratory fire hazards are potentially those that might be caused by bunsen burners and from chemicals. The most inflammable chemical commonly used is monomer. Monomer should be used in conjunction with an appropriate fume cupboard, as described earlier, and should never be used on an open bench top near to bunsen burners. All monomers should be stored in appropriate containers, clearly marked with the fire hazard signs.

Control of infection

There are two aspects to the control of infection in dentistry – cross-contamination and cross-infection. Cross-contamination may be defined as the transmission of microorganisms (pathogenic or otherwise) between patients and staff and, usually in a clinical environment, by laboratory instruments or laboratory materials. It is possible to pass infection from patient through to a dental laboratory directly. Cross-infection is the passing of infection from one person to another and may occur in any community – for example between members of the dental team or between members of a family.

In general terms cross-contamination is the aspect of infection control with which we are concerned in this section, although members of the dental team must always be alert to the possibility that they themselves may be carrying some infection which they may pass on to someone else.

The problems of cross-contamination have been highlighted in recent years due to the development of the acquired immune deficiency syndrome (AIDS). In dentistry there has been an awareness that blood and saliva are implicated in the transmission of this disease.

Whilst all aspects of dentistry are concerned with infection control this section will outline some of the problems in relation to prosthetic dentistry and dental laboratory practice. There are particular problems in this because many of the materials, instruments and procedures are difficult to handle in an infection control sense.

Organisms

There are a range of organisms that are important in dentistry, but from the dental prosthetic laboratory viewpoint two are of particular concern. These are hepatitis B virus (HBV), and human immunodeficiency virus (HIV). In addition the herpes virus is of importance when working to patient contact because it is so highly contagious.

Hepatitis B virus is a more complicated virus than HIV. Its principal actions are within the liver, but it is also found in leucocytes in all body secretions. Being present in all body fluids and strongly resistant to the usual antiseptics it is particularly dangerous. Chlorhexidine does not kill this virus, and boiling must be carried out for more than 30 minutes. Bleaching agents and ions such as fluorine and iodine or autoclaving are required. The virus may remain viable in the environment for many days.

Human immunodeficiency virus (HIV) is a much more delicate virus. Whilst it has been found in most body fluids it is easily destroyed by heat and chemical disinfectants. Antibody is produced, but the virus can exist even with this present and also retain the ability to infect.

HBV infection is more common than HIV infection, and it is difficult to diagnose in the subclinical state – thus the real incidence may be much greater than is commonly supposed. It is possible to transmit the disease via blood, semen, saliva, vaginal fluid, menses, breast milk, vomit and tears. Patients who have the acute illness are infectious whether they show symptoms of hepatitis or not. The chance of infection of a member of the dental team is much higher than with HIV. Dental surgeons and their nurses are at risk from needle-stick injuries but also from aerosol spread of infected blood and saliva. The major route of transmission to the patient is by unsterilized dental instruments.

Spread within the general population is similar to that of HIV but it may also be transmitted by biting and spitting. It is not likely that it can penetrate intact skin. About 50% of patients with HBV have subclinical infections and of the other 50% of those infected 45% show acute illness with anorexia, nausea and jaundice. There is a high morbidity and a mortality rate of 1%. A proportion of carriers continue to hold the virus and these can transmit the disease to others by most body secretions. The prevalence of the infection in dentistry may be greater than is generally believed due to the very large number of asymptomatic patients.

It may be generally accepted, in view of the frequency of occurrence of the virus, that it is important that the dentist and his team are vaccinated with the hepatitis B vaccine.

HIV patients are usually asymptomatic, and thus it is not known how many people are infected. The prevalence of HIV infection is higher in the risk group but infection by HIV does not mean that AIDS will inevitably follow.

The 'at risk' groups are homosexuals/bisexuals, intravenous drug users, persons who receive un-screened blood or blood products, and infants born to infected mothers. Needlestick injuries are a common possible source of infection, and there is some doubt as to whether AIDS can be contracted from saliva. It can be argued that, in prosthetic dentistry, in those treatments where there is no breaching of the mucosa AIDS may be considered a minimal risk when compared with the HBV infection possibilities. Herpes simplex virus causes a highly contagious vesicle on the lips during acute phases and lies dormant at other times. The vesicles shed new virus particles which are easily transmitted from person to person by physical contact through a break in the skin or mucous membrane. This virus has relevance in that the dentist may contract a lesion on the hand and this may lead to cross-infection with other members of the dental team.

Prevention

Prevention of cross-contamination and cross-infection depends upon sensible good dental practice and laboratory procedures. It is important to understand that patients infected with HBV or HIV are usually asymptomatic, and so all patients should be treated as though they are in that group. The general guidelines of good dental practice have been defined by a British Dental Association booklet and the important points are as follows.

Cleanliness

Always clean instruments and burs before sterilization.

Sterilization

Boiling is inadequate.
   Autoclave at 134°C for more than 3 minutes.
   Cold sterilizing is inadequate and should only be used if autoclaving is not possible. The procedure should be to soak in 2% glutaraldehyde for 3 hours.

Chemical sterilizing agents

There are several chemical agents that may be used for sterilization and disinfection in prosthetic dentistry but three chemicals are particularly useful.

(1) Glutaraldehyde solutions that are supplied in various sizes of container to which, in some cases, an activator must be added. It is essential to follow the manufacturers' instructions and not to exceed the shelf-life of the solution. This agent can be used for chemical soaking and items must be clean before immersion. It is not recommended as a surface disinfectant. Made-up solutions should be handled carefully as the fumes can be irritant and toxic. It should be used in a well-ventilated room.
(2) Iodophor solution is a good surface disinfectant. The chemical may be sprayed on the surface to be treated, and cleaned off using disposable paper, then resprayed and allowed to dry. This solution is not very toxic, does not have an unpleasant smell and does not irritate the skin. It may be necessary to prepare the solution each day.
(3) Bleaching agents (sodium hypochlorite) are extremely useful for cleaning down work surfaces but are not recommended as a routine disinfectant. The solution must be made up each day. It is corrosive to metals and irritant to the skin and toxic if ingested.

Equipment

Whenever possible use disposable equipment.
   Never re-use disposable equipment or needles.

Protection

Always use operating gloves. They should be worn by all staff.
   Always wash gloves with hot water and soap, detergent or special handwash solutions between patients.

Further protect cuts and abrasions under gloves with waterproof dressings.

Always wear protective glasses.

Surfaces

Where possible use sterilizable trays or disposable materials on work surfaces.

Always clean work surfaces with alcohol even though they may appear clean.

Where blood is present on a work surface clean with a disposable cloth and a hypochlorite solution (glutaraldehyde if metal) or a cleaner containing a hypochlorite.

Waste

All sharp cutting instruments should also be placed into an approved container. All other items should be placed in stout plastic bags, sealed and incinerated.

The cycle of possible infection in dental prosthetics passes from the patient to dental surgeon to dental nurse to dental technician and back again. The procedures that are recommended must, therefore, break that cycle at each point to ensure that cross-contamination and cross-infection cannot occur.

The cycle of care begins with the dental surgeon and his nurse protecting themselves and by adequate control of the state of the instruments to be used and the actual procedures. It is important that each clinical prosthetic stage is thought through and the appropriate instruments used. For example, it is necessary to use metal rulers and not plastic rulers. Pressure indicating paste should not be applied with a paint brush which is then re-used and wooden-handled instruments are not satisfactory.

It is important that prosthetic work for the laboratory should be decontaminated before leaving the clinic.

The general procedures that should be adopted are as follows:

(1) Silicone impression materials should be used for impressions and disposable trays for primary impressions or in any case where special trays have not been prescribed. These impressions should be washed in running tap water then placed in a container with 2% glutaraldehyde solution for at least 30 minutes. They should then be rewashed and placed in a sealed polythene bag before being sent to the laboratory. On receipt in the laboratory they should be soaked for a further 3 hours, although this is not necessary if the longer 3-hour soak is completed at the clinic. Labelling is important so that the laboratory can be aware of the procedures that have been completed up to the time of dispatch.

Alginate impressions are not advised as sterilization can be difficult. If soaked in bleaching agents they will distort, and so they should be washed, sprayed with iodophor, rinsed again, sprayed with iodophor and sealed in a polythene bag.

(2) The cycle of contamination should be broken in the clinic for other items of prosthetic work, and so a decontamination procedure must apply to any item that has come from the patient's mouth. This includes any denture and try-in. These items of work should be thoroughly washed, cleaned of all debris, blood and saliva, and decontaminated. Decontamination should be carried out as described above for silicone impressions.

(3) Prostheses that require adjustment should not be removed to the laboratory or any other area. Any necessary procedure should be completed at the chairside, thus containing the activity to the operating area. This has the advantage of constricting the zone of contamination.

(4) In the laboratory that receives prosthetic work from practitioners the procedure that has been completed must be clearly indicated. There are restrictions on the sending of infected matter by the postal services, and so all work dispatched by the Royal Mail Services must be decontaminated. As indicated above this should apply to all work that leaves the clinic, but if there is any doubt the laboratory should treat the work as infected upon arrival. If infection is suspected the dental technician unpacking the work should be gloved, masked and wear spectacles. The decontamination procedure that should be followed is that already described for silicone impressions earlier. After unpacking work from the clinic, where full decontamination is not guaranteed, all packaging should be destroyed. It is important to recognize that casts can be infected from impressions, and so ideally decontamination of impressions must be thoroughly completed before the impressions are poured. Casts may be decontaminated, if that is thought to be necessary, by spraying with iodophor. Work leaving the laboratory should also be washed and disinfected before dispatch.

(5) Decontamination procedures for prostheses will depend upon whether metal is present. Prostheses not containing metal may be soaked in dilute hypochlorite solution for 10 minutes. Metal prostheses may be soaked in chlorhexidine digluconate (Hibiscrub) or undiluted iodophor.

Frequent changing of polishing agents – such as pumice troughs – is essential to reduce cross-contamination and technicians should use glasses and face masks when polishing. It is essential that the filtration systems on the grinding and polishing machines are functioning satisfactorily.

Polishing attachments can be sterilized successfully. Brushes should be washed and soaked for 3 hours in 2% glutaraldehyde. Mops and fabric polishing wheels should be washed and autoclaved, and metal cutters and stones should be cleaned manually, then ultrasonically and then sterilized chemically.

Transport of work between laboratory and the clinic, should be by means of a sealed plastic bag and disposable trays should be used for larger items.

All disposable items should be placed in the appropriate plastic bag and incinerated.

Vaccination

It is advisable for all members of the dental team to be vaccinated against hepatitis B (HBV).

Bibliography

General

Applegate, O. C. (1965) *The Essentials of Removable Partial Denture Prostheses,* 3rd edition, Saunders, Philadelphia

Basker, R. M., Davenport, J. C. and Tomlin, H. R. (1983) *Prosthetic Treatment of the Edentulous Patient,* 2nd edition, Macmillan Press, London

Basker, R., Harrison, A. and Ralph, J. P. (1988) *Overdentures in General Dental Practice,* BDA Publication, London

Bates, J. F., Adams, D. and Stafford, G. D. (1984) *Dental Treatment of the Elderly,* Wright, Bristol

Beresin, V. E. and Schiesser, F. J. (1978) *The Neutral Zone in Complete Dentures,* 2nd edition, Mosby, St Louis, MO

Blakeslee, R. W., Renner, R. P. and Shiu, A. (1980) *Dental Technology Theory and Practice,* C. V. Mosby Co., St Louis, MO

Brecker, S. C. (1966) *Clinical Procedures in Occlusal Rehabilitation,* Saunders, Philadelphia and London

Combe, E. C. (1981) *Notes on Dental Materials,* 4th edition, Churchill Livingstone, Edinburgh

Dental Technician Prosthetic (1962) US Navy Training Course, Bureau of Naval Personnel, Superintendent of Documents, US Government Printing Office, Washington DC

Heartwell, C. M. and Rahn, A. O. (1980) *Syllabus of Complete Dentures,* 3rd edition, Lee and Febiger, Philadelphia

Hickey, J. C., Zarb, G. A. and Bolender, C. L. (1985) *Boucher's Prosthodontic Treatment for Edentulous Patients,* 9th edition, C. V. Mosby Co., St Louis, MO

Krol, A. J. (1981) *Removable Partial Dentures Design,* University of the Pacific, San Francisco

McGivney, G. P. and Castleberry, D. J. (1989) *MacCrackens Removable Partial Prosthodontics,* 8th edition. Mosby, St Louis

Morrow, R. M., Rudd, K. D. and Rhoads, J. E. (1986) *Dental Laboratory Procedures, Complete Dentures,* Vol. 1, C. V. Mosby Co., St Louis, MO

Preiskel, H. W. (1973) *Precision Attachments in Dentistry,* Kimpton, London

Pullen-Warner, E. and L'Estrange, P. R. (1978) *Sectional Dentures – A Simplified Method of Attachment,* Wright, Bristol

Sears, V. H. (1949) *Principles and Techniques for Complete Denture Construction,* C. V. Mosby Co., St Louis, MO

Sowter, J. B. (1968) *Dental Laboratory Technology,* The University of North Carolina Press, Chapel Hill, NC

Watt, D. M. and MacGregor, A. R. (1976) *Designing Complete Dentures,* Saunders, Philadelphia

Zarb, G. A., Bergman, B. O., Clayton, J. A. and MacKay, H. F. (1978) *Prosthodontic Treatment for Partially Edentulous Patients,* C. V. Mosby, St Louis, MO

Chapter 1

Applegate, O. C. (1957) Conditions which will influence the choice of partial or complete denture service. *J. Pros. Dent.,* 7, 182

Beyron, H. L. (1964) Characteristics of functionally optimal occlusion and principles of occlusal rehabilitation. *J. Am. Dent. Assoc.,* 48, 648

Fish, S. H. (1969) Adaption and habituation to full dentures. *Br. Dent. J.,* 127, 19

Green, J. C. and Vermillion, J. R. (1964) The Simplified Oral Hygiene Index. *J. Am. Dent. Assoc.,* **68**, 7

Ramjford, S. P. (1959) Indices for prevalence and incidence of periodontal diseases. *J. Periodontol.,* **30**, 51

Chapter 2

Christiansen, R. L. (1959) The rationale of the facebow in maxillary cast mountings. *J. Prosth. Dent.,* **9**, 388

Lawson, W. A. (1978) Current concepts and practice in complete dentures. Impressions: principles and practice. *J. Dent.,* **6**, 43

Chapter 3

Air Force Manual 160-29 (1959) *Dental Laboratory Technician's Manual,* United States Air Force, Washington DC, p. 101

Sharry, J. J. (1974) *Complete Denture Prosthodontics,* 3rd edition, McGraw-Hill Book Co., New York, p. 211

Chapter 4

Harris, L. W. (1960) Boxing and cast pouring. *J. Prosth. Dent.,* **10**, 390

Chapter 5

Frush, J. P. and Fisher, R. D. (1958) The dynesthetic interpretation of the dentogenic concept. *J. Prosth. Dent.,* **8**, 558

Lee, J. (1962) *Aesthetics,* J. Wright, Bristol

Monteith, B. (1984) The role of the freeway space in the generation of muscle pain among denture wearers. *J. Oral Rehab.,* **11**, 483

Potgeiter, P. J., Monteith, B. and Kemp, P. L. (1983) The determination of freeway space in edentulous patients: a cephlomatric approach. *J. Oral Rehabil.,* **10**, 283

Pound, E. (1960) Modern American concepts of aesthetics, *Int. Dent. J.,* **10**, 154

Tryde, G., MacMillan, D. R., Christiensen, J. and Brill, N. (1976) The fallacy of facial measurements of occlusal height in edentulous subjects. *J. Oral Rehabil.,* **3**, 353

Chapter 6

Humphrey, J., Murphy, W. M. and Huggett, R. (1979) Mounting casts onto articulators. *Dent. Techn.,* **32**, 2, 4

Murphy, W. M. and Huggett, R. (1978) Articulators in complete denture construction. *Dent. Techn.,* **37**, 6

Chapter 7

Heath, R. (1970) A study of the morphology of the denture space. *Dent. Pract.,* **21**, 109

Mehringer, E. J. (1963) Use of speech patterns as an aid in prosthodontic reconstruction. *J. Prosth. Dent.,* **13**, 825

Monson, G. S. (1922) Some important factors which influence occlusion. *J. Nat. Dent. Assoc.,* **9**, 498–502

Neill, D. J. and Glaysher, J. K. L. (1982) Identifying the denture space. *J. Oral Rehabil.,* **9**, 259

Smith, R. A., Cavalcanti, A. A. and Wolfe, H. E. (1986) Arranging and articulating artificial teeth. In *Dental Laboratory Procedures, Complete Dentures* (ed. R. M. Morrow, K. D. Rudd and J. E. Rhoads), C. V. Mosby Co., St Louis, MO, pp. 223–275

Tallgren, A. (1972) Continuing reduction of the residual alveolar ridges in complete denture wearers: a mixed longitudinal study covering 25 years. *J. Prosth. Dent.,* **27**, 120

Watt, D. M. and Likeman, P. R. (1974) Morphological changes in the denture bearing areas following the extraction of maxillary teeth. *Br. Dent. J.,* **136**, 225

Wright, C. R. (1966) Evaluation of the factors necessary to develop stability in mandibular dentures. *J. Prosth. Dent.,* **16**, 414

Chapter 8

Becker, C. M. and Bolender, C. L. (1981) Designing swing lock partial dentures. *J. Prosth. Dent.,* **46**, 126

Beckett, L. S. (1953) The influence of saddle classification on the design of partial removable restorations. *J. Prosth. Dent.,* **3**, 506

Bennett, N. G. (1958) A contribution to the study of the movements of the mandible. *J. Prosth. Dent.,* **8**, 41

Farrell, J. H. (1956) The effect of mastication on the digestion of food. *Br. Dent. J.,* **100**, 149

Johnston, J. W. (1958) All acrylic partial dentures. *N. Z. Dent. J.,* **54**, 67

Krol, A. J. and Finzen, F. C. (1989) Rotational path removable partial dentures. Part 1. Replacement of posterior teeth. *Int. J. Prosth.,* **1**, 17

Chapter 10

Anderson, J. N. (1958) Dimensions of casts palatal and lingual bars. *Dent. Pract.*, **7**, 270

Basker, R. M. and Tryde, G. (1977) Connectors for mandibular partial dentures. Use of the sublingual bar. *J. Oral Rehab.*, **4**, 389

Blatterfein, L. (1951) Study of partial denture clasping. *J. Am. Dent. Ass.*, **43**, 169

Brill, N., Tryde, G., Stoltze, A. and Ghamrawy El, E. A. (1977) The ecological changes in oral cavity caused by removable partial dentures. *J. Prosth. Dent.*, **38**, 138

Campbell, L. D. (1977) Subjective reactions to major connector designs for removable dentures. *J. Prosth. Dent.*, **37**, 507

Cummer, W. E. (1942) *The American Textbook of Prosthetic Dentistry* 7th edition (ed. L. Pierce Anthony), Henry Kimpton, London, Chapter XVI

Demer, W. J. (1976) An analysis of the mesial rest – I bar clasp designs. *J. Prosth. Dent.*, **36**, 243

Frank, R. P. and Nicholls, J. I. (1977) An investigation of the effectiveness of indirect retainers. *J. Prosth. Dent.*, **38**, 494

Nairn, R. I. (1966) The problem of free end denture bases. *J. Prosth. Dent.*, **16**, 522

Scally, K. B. (1988) The 'Every' partial denture system: the mandibular partial denture. *N. Z. Dent. Ass. Prosthodont. J.*, **7**, 19

Steffel, V. L. (1951) Fundamental principles in partial denture design with special reference to equalization of tooth and tissue support. *Dent. J. Aust.*, **23**, 68

Wagner, G. A. and Traweek, F. C. (1982) Comparison of major connector for removable partial dentures. *J. Prosth. Dent.*, **47**, 242

Waters, N. E. (1972) The rigidity of lingual bars. *Dent. Pract.*, **22**, 209

Chapter 11

Beyron, H. L. (1954) Occlusal changes in the adult dentition. *J. Am. Dent. Assoc.*, **48**, 674

Graham, C. H. (1953) Occlusal correction. *Dent. J. Aust.*, **25**, 181

MacCracken, W. L. (1956) Mouth preparation for partial dentures. *J. Prosth. Dent.*, **6**, 39

Chapter 12

Bates, J. F. (1965) The mechanical properties of cobalt chromium alloys and their relation to partial denture design. *Br. Dent. J.*, **119**, 389

Bates, J. F. (1968) Studies in retention of cobalt chromium partial dentures. *Br. Dent. J.*, **125**, 97

Lorton, L. (1978) A method of stabilizing removable partial denture castings during clinical and laboratory procedures. *J. Prosth. Dent.*, **39**, 344

Chapter 13

Beckett, L. S. (1954) Accurate occlusal relations in partial denture construction. *J. Prosth. Dent.*, **4**, 487

Ellinger, C. W., Somes, G. W., Nicholl, B. R., Unger, J. W. and Wesley, R. C. (1979) Patient response to variations in denture technique. Part III. Five year subjective evaluation. *J. Prosth. Dent.*, **42**, 127

Grant, A. A. (1962) The effect of the investment procedure on tooth movement. *J. Prosth. Dent.*, **12**, 1053

Grant, A. A. (1963) Elevation of the incisal guide pin following attachment of cast to articulators. *J. Prosth. Dent.*, **13**, 664

Nicol, B. R., Somes, G. W., Ellinger, C. W., Unger, J. W. and Fuhrmann, J. (1979) Patient response to variations in denture technique. Part II. *J. Prosth. Dent.*, **41**, 368

Sidhaye, A. B. and Master, S. B. (1979) Efficacy of remount procedures using masticatory performance tests. *J. Prosth. Dent.*, **41**, 129

Wesley, R. C., Ellinger, C. W. and Somes, G. W. (1984) Patient response to variations in denture techniques. Part VI. Mastication of peanuts and carrots. *J. Prosth. Dent.*, **51**, 467

Chapter 14

Huggett, R., Brooks, S. C. and Bates, J. F. (1985) Which curing cycle is best. *Dent. Techn., (Techn. Suppl.)*, **38**, 11

Jerolimov, V., Huggett, R., Brooks, S. C. and Bates, J. F. (1985) The effect of variations in the polymer/monomer mixing ratios on residual monomer levels and flexural properties of denture base materials. *Quint. Dent. Techn.*, **9**, 431

Wright, P. S. (1976) Soft lining materials: their status and prospects. *J. Dent.*, **4**, 247

Chapter 15

Rudd, D. D., Morrow, R. M., Espinoza, A. V. and Leachman, J. S. (1986) Finishing and Polishing. In *Dental Laboratory Procedures, Complete Dentures* (ed. R. M. Morrow, K. D. Rudd and J. E. Rhoads), C. V. Mosby Co., St Louis, MO

Chapter 16

Bassiouny, M. A. and Grant, A. A. (1975) The toothbrush application of chlorhexidine. *Br. Dent. J.,* **139**, 323

Rantanen, T., Siirila, H. S. and Lehvila, P. (1979) The effect of instruction and motivation on dental knowledge and behaviour among partial denture wearers. *Odont. Scand.,* **38**, 9

Chapter 17

Fish, S. F. (1969) Adaptation and habituation to full dentures. *Br. Dent. J.,* **127**, 19

Gillings, B. R. D. (1981) Magnetic retention for complete and partial overdentures, *J. Prosth. Dent.,* **45**, 484 and 607

Robinson, J. G. (1976) A denture copying technique when providing replacement dentures. *J. Dent.,* **4**, 15

Stafford, G. D. and Huggett, R. (1971) The use of duplicate dentures in complete denture construction. *Dent. Pract. Dent. Rec.,* **22**, 119

Appendix IV

Atkinson, H. F. (1953) Partial dentures problems: designing about a path of withdrawal. *Aust. J. Dent.,* **57**, 187

Craddock, F. W. (1955) Clasp surveying and mysticism. *Aust. J. Dent.,* **59**, 205

Craddock, F. W. and Bottomley, G. A. (1954) Second thoughts on clasp surveying. *Br. Dent. J.,* **96**, 134

Appendix V

Barbenel, J. C. (1971) Physical retention of complete dentures. *J. Prosth. Dent.,* **26**, 592

Brill, N. (1967) Factors in the mechanism of full denture retention – discussion of selective papers. *Dent. Pract.,* **18**, 9

Kawazoe, Y. and Hamada, T. (1978) The role of saliva in retention of maxillary complete dentures. *J. Prosth. Dent.,* **40**, 131

Lindstrom, R. E., Pawelchak, J., Heyd, A. and Tarbet, W. J. (1979) Physical-chemical aspects of denture retention and stability: a review of the literature. *J. Prosth. Dent.,* **42**, 371

Roydhouse, R. H. (1960) Retention of dentures. *J. Amer. Dent. Ass.,* **60**, 159

Russell, A. L. (1956) A system of classification and scoring for prevalence surveys of periodontal disease. *J. Dent. Res.,* **35**, 352

Stanitz, J. D. (1948) An analysis of the part played by the fluid film in denture retention. *J. Am. Dent. Assoc.,* **37**, 168

Stephan, M. J. (1874) Versuche uber scheinbare adhasion sitzungsberichte der Kaiserlichen. *Akad. Wissench Vienna Mathematisch-Naturwissen Schaftiche Klasse,* **69**, 713

Product directories

The Dental Practice Directory (1990) A. E. Morgan Publications Ltd, Stanley House, 9 West Street, Epsom KT18 7RL, Surrey

The Dental Technician Yearbook and Directory (1990) A. E. Morgan Publications Ltd, Stanley House, 9 West Street, Epsom KT18 7RL, Surrey

Glossary

Bonwill, W. G. A. (1885) Geometrical and mechanical laws of articulation. *Tr. Odontological Society of Pennsylvania,* **119**, 133

British Standard Glossary of Dental Terms (1983) BS4492, British Standards Institution, London

Glossary of Prosthodontic Terms (1977) The Academy of Denture Prosthetics, C. V. Mosby Co., St Louis, MO

Spee, F. von (1890) Die Verschiebungsbahn des Unterkiefers am Schädel. *Arch. für Anat. und Physiol.*

Glossary of prosthodontic terms

A universal acceptance of a standard terminology is essential to clear understanding of any subject. Agreed formal glossaries are now part of the literature of prosthetic dentistry both in the United Kingdom and in the United States of America. Specialist societies have participated in the preparation of the glossaries as they appreciate that communication is impossible without generally agreed scientific terminology.

Some of the technical terms used in this book are set out in this section and are taken from the *British Standard Glossary of Dental Terms* (BS4492:1983) to whom we are grateful for permission to publish. It is not a comprehensive list of all terms used in prosthetic dentistry and has been restricted to those terms expected to occur with reasonable frequency. In some cases, where two or more terms have the same meaning, the first listed term is preferred.

Term	Definition
Abutment	A tooth, root, or portion of an implant used for the support or anchorage of a fixed or removable prosthesis.
Adhesion	The physical force that attracts certain dissimilar molecules when in close approximation.
Adjustable axis facebow Hinge axis locating facebow	A device, with adjustable side arms, that is attached to the mandible and used to locate the retruded hinge axis. Mandibular opening and closing movements are made in retruded jaw relation and the condyle pointers are adjusted until they rotate without translation.
Acrylic polymer Acrylic resin	A general term for synthetic polymers in which the repeating unit is a derivative of acrylic acid, usually methyl methacrylate. Polymerization is effected by a free radical mechanism which may be produced by heat energy, light energy, or chemical means. Systems using chemical means include those known as autopolymerizing, cold-curing, rapid-curing. The principal use is in the fabrication of dentures and synthetic resin teeth.
Agar impression material	A reversible hydrocolloid impression material consisting of an aqueous agar gel. It liquefies when heated and returns to the gel state on cooling.
Ala–tragal line Camper's plane	The line running from the inferior border of the ala of the nose to the superior border of the tragus of the ear.
Alginate impression material	An irreversible hydrocolloid impression material in which a powder, consisting of soluble alginates and additives, is mixed with water and which on setting forms a gel. Gel formation is achieved by the precipitation of an insoluble calcium salt.

Arrow-point tracing
Gothic arch tracing
A horizontal tracing which resembles an arrowhead or a gothic arch, made by a tracer, and representing the posterior border movement of the mandible.

Articulating paper
A strip of paper or cellulose acetate sheet coated with pigment used for marking areas of contact between opposing teeth.

Attachment
A colloquial synonym for precision attachment.

Autopolymerizing
Self-cure
Cold-cure
Any resin that will polymerize with an activator and initiator but without the use of external heat.

Balanced occlusion
Simultaneous contacts of the occluding surfaces on both sides of the mouth, in various jaw positions.

Baseplate
The foundation on which an occlusal rim is built or on which a trial denture is set up.

Bennett angle
The angle between the sagittal plane and the path of the advancing condyle during lateral mandibular movement, as viewed along the horizontal plane.

Bennett movement
The lateral translation of the mandible during lateral exertion.

Bite registration material
Occlusal indicator wax
Bite wax
A material used to register occlusion between opposing faces of maxillary and mandibular teeth. It is usually in the form of a wax or a paste.

Bonwill triangle
A 4-inch (102 mm) equilateral triangle postulated by Bonwill, formed by the medial contact of the mandibular central incisors and the centres of the condyles.

Border moulding
The shaping of an impression material by the manipulation or activity of the soft tissues adjacent to the borders of an impression.

Border movement
A movement of the mandible along the extremity of its range, in any direction.

Border seal
The contact between the denture border and the adjacent tissues which prevents the passage of air.

Boxing
Of an impression. The provision of a wall, usually in wax, attached to the perimeter of an impression, in order to contain the cast material until it is set.

Boxing wax
A wax that will adhere to impression material and is used to form a mould into which laboratory plaster or dental stone can be poured.

Bracing arm
See reciprocating arm.

Cast
(1) (Noun). A reproduction of the surface form of oral or facial tissues obtained from an impression.
(2) (Verb). To form a cast from an impression or to form a casting in a mould.

Casting
An object, usually of metal, formed in a mould.

Christiansen's phenomenon
The development of a gap between the posterior ends of opposing flat occlusal rims, which occurs when the mandible is protruded.

Cohesion
The property of a material by which its constituent molecules are attracted to each other and resist separation.

Compensating curve
The curvature of the occlusal plane of dentures, created to permit balanced occlusion. The curve compensates for the effects of Christiansen's phenomenon.

Condylar angle
The angle between the sagittal projection of the condylar path and the Frankfurt plane.

Condylar guide
That part of an articulator which guides its condylar element, approximately as the mandibular joint guides the condyle.

Condylar guide angle
The angle of inclination of the condylar guide to the horizontal plane or other reference plane.

Condylar path	Any path travelled by the mandibular condyle during the various mandibular movements.
Copy dentures Replica dentures Duplicate dentures	Copies of the patient's dentures that are used in the construction of new dentures.
Coronal plane	Any plane passing longitudinally through the body from side to side, at right angles to the mid-sagittal plane, and dividing the body into front and back parts.
Curve of Monson Monson's curve	The curve of occlusion of natural teeth, described by Monson, in which each cusp and incisal edge touches or conforms to a segment of the surface of a sphere 4 inches (102 mm) in radius with its centre in the region of the glabella. *Note.* It is commonly assumed that this curve is an arch viewed only from the front of the mouth.
Curve of Spee	An arc of a circle of 65 mm to 70 mm radius, described by Spee, that touches the tips of all the mandibular teeth when the skull is viewed laterally. When continued, it touches the anterior surface of the condyles.
Cusp angle	An angle made by the slopes of the cusp with the plane perpendicular to the long axis of the tooth.
Dental articulation Articulation	The close approximation of, or contact between, opposing teeth that occurs while the mandible is moving.
Denture base	That part of the denture that rests on the denture-bearing area of the oral mucosa.
Denture base material	A material, usually composed of an acrylic polymer bead and acrylic monomer, used in the construction of dentures and other appliances by a dough-moulding technique.
Diagnostic cast Study cast	A cast as an aid to diagnosis and treatment planning.

Direct retainer	A component of a partial denture that resists dislodgement along the path of withdrawal.
Direct retention	The retention obtained in a partial denture by the use of direct retainers.
Doughing time	That part of the working time measured from the end of the mixing time until the time a material is ready for manipulation. It is generally used in connection with denture base resins and acrylic resin teeth.
Duplicating material Agar duplicating material	A material used in the dental laboratory to duplicate accurately models, casts or other items. It is usually based on a hydrocolloid impression material such as agar or alginate.
Eccentric jaw relation	Any jaw relation that is lateral or protrusive to the retruded jaw relation.
Eccentric occlusion	Any occlusion that is not the intercuspal occlusion.
Elastomeric impression material	An impression material based on a non-aqueous polymeric system which exhibits rubber-like behaviour. The most important types are based on silicones, polysulphides and polyethers.
Endosteal implant Endosseus implant	An implant, usually made of metal, which is inserted into the edentulous alveolar bone so that part protrudes into the mouth. The protruding end is used as an attachment for a prosthesis.
Envelope of movement	The three-dimensional space circumscribed by border movements of a given point in the mandible (or a device rigidly attached to it).
Extracoronal attachment	A presision attachment joined to a restoration and situated outside the coronal contour.
Extra-oral tracing	An arrow-point tracing made outside the oral cavity.
Facebow	An instrument used to record the relation of the maxilla to the hinge axis of rotation of the mandible. It enables a

	similar relation to be established between the maxillary casts and the hinge axis of the articulator.
Final impression Master impression Working impression Second impression	The impression that is used for making the master cast. *Note.* 'Second impression' refers specifically to the final impression. There is no such term as third, etc., impression.
Flask	(1) (Noun). A sectional metal case that contains and supports the mould in which dentures are formed. (2) (Verb). To invest the pattern in the flask.
Frankfurt plane	A plane passing through the lowest point in the floor of the left orbit, and the highest point in the margin of each external auditory meatus of the skull. It approximates to the horizontal when the head is in a normal upright position.
Functional impression	An impression that during its formation is modified by masticatory loads and adjacent muscular activity. *Note.* See also mucodisplacement impression.
Gingivally-approaching clasp Roach clasp	A clasp, whose terminal point approaches a tooth from the direction of the gingivae.
Gnathodynamometer	An instrument for measuring the force exerted in closing the jaws.
Grinding-in	Occlusal correction of artificial teeth by grinding.
Guide plane	Two or more paralleled surfaces of abutment teeth prepared to limit the path of insertion and improve the stability of a removable prosthesis.
High-impact denture base material	A denture base material formulated to have higher resistance to fracture by impact or fatigue.
High lip-line	The greatest height to which the upper lip is normally raised in function.

Hinge axis	A horizontal axis in the region of the condyles about which the mandible can rotate without translatory movement of the condyles.
Horizontal overlap Overjet	A projection of the maxillary teeth beyond the mandibular teeth in the horizontal plane.
Hydrocolloid impression material	A general term used to refer to alginate and agar impression materials. Chemically, these are colloidal materials with water initially as the dispersing phase. After gelation, water becomes the disperse phase.
Impression compound Compound	A thermoplastic material used to take impressions, comprising natural and synthetic resins, fillers and plasticizers, in the form of sticks, sheets and cones. It is softened to a working consistency by immersion in hot water or by warming over a flame.
Impression plaster	Finely ground plaster of Paris containing additives (e.g. potassium sulphate and borax) that minimize setting expansion and control the setting time.
Incisal angle	The angle formed with the horizontal plane by drawing a line in the sagittal plane between the incisal edges of the maxillary and mandibular central incisors when the teeth are in intercuspal occlusion.
Incisal guidance	The guidance provided by the surfaces of the maxillary incisors in lateral movement of the mandible.
Incisal guide Incisal table	That part of an articulator which maintains the incisal angle.
Incisal guide angle	The angle to which the incisal guide is set.
Indirect retention	The retention obtained by the extension of a partial denture base to provide the fulcrum of a class II lever. The retainer(s) providing direct retention lie between the fulcrum and that part of the denture which is subject to the displacing force.

Infra-orbital pointer Infra-orbital indicator	The component of a facebow that records infra-orbital notch position and thereby aligns it with the Frankfurt plane.
Interalveolar distance Inter-ridge distance	The vertical distance between specified positions on the maxillary and mandibular alveolar ridges at the vertical dimension of occlusion.
Intercuspal occlusion Centric occlusion	Maximal contact between opposing teeth.
Intercuspal position	The position of the mandible when the teeth are in intercuspal occlusion.
Intercuspation	The interdigitation of cusps of opposing teeth.
Interocclusal	Between opposing occlusal surfaces.
Interocclusal space Freeway space	The space between the maxillary and mandibular occluding surfaces when the mandible is in the rest position.
Interocclusal record	A record of any relation of opposing occlusal surfaces. *Note.* It is essential to specify the type of record, e.g. intercuspal, retrusive, protrusive or lateral, and contact or pre-contact.
Intracoronal attachment	A precision attachment, one part of which is totally embedded in a restoration.
Master cast Final cast	The cast produced from the final impression.
Modelling wax	A blend of waxes, usually pink, red or orange in colour, that is adaptable at ambient temperature. The softening temperature range varies according to the intended use.
Mucodisplacement impression	An impression made with the intention of displacing soft tissues. *Note.* See also functional impression.
Mucostatic impression	An impression made with the intention of minimizing mucosal displacement.
Neutral zone	A term used to describe a zone in which the opposing forces of the cheeks/lips and tongue are said to be in equilibrium.
Non-working side Balancing side Contralateral side	The side opposite the working side.
Non-working side contacts Balancing contacts	The contacts between maxillary and mandibular teeth, or denture bases on the non-working side, or posteriorly in a protrusive occlusion.
Occlusal plane Plane of occlusion	An imaginary surface that touches the incisal surfaces of the maxillary incisors and the tips of the cusps of the posterior teeth. This surface is usually curved and is not strictly a plane.
Occlusal rim Occlusion rim	An occluding surface formed of mouldable material which is attached to a temporary or permanent denture base, for the purpose of recording jaw relations and indicating tooth positions.
Occlusal vertical dimension Occlusal face height	Any vertical dimension when the teeth or occlusal rims are in contact.
Occlusally-approaching clasp	A clasp originating from the occlusal side of the survey line.
Occlusion	Any contact between teeth of opposing dental arches, usually referring to contact between the occlusal surface.
Packing	The act of filling a mould with a plastic material in order to construct a dental prosthesis.
Pantograph	A complex of tracing devices attached to the mandible and maxilla which enables records of mandibular movements to be made in three planes.
Path of insertion/ withdrawal	The path followed by the denture from its first contact with the supporting tissues until it is fully seated.
Polished surface	The surface of the denture, usually polished, which is in contact with the lips, cheeks and tongue, excluding the occlusal surfaces.

Polyether impression material	An impression material based on an organic polymer in which the repeating unit contains an ether linkage. Setting is achieved by the cross-linking reaction of pendant ethylene-imino groups, activated by acidic catalysts.
Poly(methyl methacrylate) (PMMA)	An acrylic polymer, formed by the polymerization of methyl methacrylate and widely used for the fabrication of denture bases and acrylic resin teeth, by the dough technique.
Polysulphide impression material	An impression material based on an organic polymer in which the repeating units are linked by disulphide groups. They are often referred to as mercaptans or thiokols. Setting is commonly achieved by increase in chain length and cross-linking.
Posterior palatal seal	The seal at the posterior border of a maxillary denture.
Post-dam	A ridge of denture base material on the posterior border of the maxillary denture impression surface which displaces the supporting soft tissues in order to create a seal.
Precision attachment	A prefabricated interlocking device, one component of which is fixed to an abutment while the other is integrated into a denture or bridge in order to support and/or retain it.
Process Cure	A procedure whereby denture base resin is polymerized in a mould.
Pourable denture base material Pour resin Pourable resin Pour-type resin	A denture base material specially formulated to allow it to flow under gravity to fill a mould.
Radio-opaque denture base material	A denture base material rendered opaque to X-rays by the inclusion of a radio-opaque material to facilitate location in human tissues.
Rebase	The removal and replacement of the denture base.
Reciprocating arm	A component of a partial denture used to prevent displacement of a tooth by a direct retainer.
Reline	The addition of material to the existing surface of a denture base.
Rest jaw relation	The relation of the mandible to the maxilla when the mandible is in the rest position.
Rest vertical dimension	The vertical dimension with the mandible in the rest position.
Retruded jaw relation Centric jaw relation Centric relation	Any position of the mandible on its retruded arc of closure.
Sectional impression	An impression built up in the mouth from two or more parts which are then removed separately and reassembled.
Selective grinding Spot grinding	The planned adjustment of the occlusal forms of teeth by grinding with a stone.
Separating medium	A material used to facilitate the separation of a plaster surface from another surface of plaster, or other material (notably impression materials and denture base resins), and prevent or reduce the transfer of moisture. Alginates are the most widely-used materials for this purpose.
Silicone impression material	An impression material based on an organo-siloxane polymer, with silicon–oxygen links form the basic structure. Setting is achieved by cross-linking induced by various catalyst systems.
Soft liner Resilient liner	A soft, polymeric material used on the fitting surfaces of dentures to reduce trauma to the soft supporting tissues. They are generally synthetic elastomers or plasticized acrylic polymers.
Special tray Custom tray	An impression tray made specifically for an individual patient by means of which the impression material may be accurately controlled.

Split mounting

A method of mounting the cast on an articulator to facilitate removal and accurate replacement. It may also be used for checking the accuracy of jaw relation records.

Sticky wax

A blend of waxes that, when heated, melts and adheres to the surfaces to which it is applied. Its primary purpose is to hold components together prior to permanent fixation.

Synthetic resin teeth
Acrylic resin teeth

Artificial teeth fabricated from synthetic resin. The resin most commonly used is poly(methyl methacrylate).

Tissue conditioner

A specialized type of soft liner, used for short duration, which is intended to improve the condition of the soft tissues supporting the prosthesis. It is usually a highly plasticized acrylic polymer.

Tracing stick

An impression compound in stick form, having a low softening point and used mainly for adapting the margins of impressions trays, or for taking inlay/crown impressions.

Trial denture
Try-in

The arrangement of teeth in wax for trial insertion prior to completion of the denture.

Tray adhesive

A material for ensuring adhesion between the impression material and the containing tray. These are often specific to the type of impression material concerned, e.g. polysulphide adhesive.

Veined denture base material

A denture base material to which short threads made of nylon, or other suitable organic filaments are added to simulate the appearance of blood vessels.

Vertical overlap overbite

The extension of the maxillary teeth over the mandibular teeth in a vertical direction when the opposing teeth are in the intercuspal position.

Working time

The period of time, measured from the start of mixing, during which it is possible to manipulate a dental material without an adverse effect on its properties. Working time comprises mixing time, doughing time (when appropriate) and manipulation time. *Note.* This is the 'normal' definition. Variations do exist in certain standards.

Zinc oxide–eugenol impression paste

An impression paste obtained by mixing two pastes, one containing zinc oxide together with an oil such as liquid paraffin and an accelerator such as zinc acetate, and the other containing a resin such as colophony dissolved in eugenol.

Index